Praise
Movement for

MW00562417

"*Movement for Every Body* is the perfect book and guide for anyone with a body. It's accessible, insightful, and practical. This book breaks down all the barriers to movement, while giving readers the tools and skills to put what they're reading into practice in actionable and meaningful ways. I highly recommend this book to anyone who engages in movement as well as movement practitioners of all backgrounds."

—CHRISSY KING, author of *The Body Liberation Project*

"Somehow, Dr. Marcia has transmuted a career's worth of knowledge and wisdom into a practical, actionable guide for taking care of your human body in a complicated world. I want to have this book near me when I'm journaling, when I'm working out, when I'm in therapy, when I'm working with clients . . . it should be required reading for anyone who is starting out on their journey to a happier relationship with fitness and movement!"

—LAURA GIRARD, CPT, founder of The Energy Academy

"In a world where fitness advice can feel very loud and extremely exclusive, *Movement for Every Body* provides a calm, welcoming presence. The book tackles complex topics with a kindness and confidence that genuinely considers a variety of experiences. Not only does the book tap into so many nuances when it comes to participating in exercise, but it also includes a plethora of options and examples to help folks explore as they go. Whether you have been working out for years or you are just getting started, if you are interested in cultivating a more accessible and joyful relationship with movement, you'll definitely want to read this book."

—LAUREN LEAVELL, NASM-certified personal trainer and barre teacher

"Through *Movement for Every Body,* Dr. Marcia creates a robust and inclusive invitation that allows one to explore why they believe what they do about movement in relation to their own bodies and others. Then she provides the necessary tools to help one rebuild their relationship with movement, all while keeping accessibility at the forefront. If your relationship to health and movement is strained, and you want to restore the joy in your health journey, this is a perfect place to begin."

—DR. JENNIFER D. HUTTON, physical therapist and creator of *The Get Movin' Activity Deck* and the *Beyond Allyship* podcast

Movement
for
Every Body

An Inclusive Fitness Guide
for Better Movement

Marcia Dernie, DPT

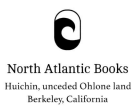

North Atlantic Books
Huichin, unceded Ohlone land
Berkeley, California

Published by
North Atlantic Books
Huichin, unceded Ohlone land
Berkeley, California

Cover and interior photos © Bianca Valentim Photography
Cover design by Jess Morphew
Book design by Happenstance Type-O-Rama

Printed in the United States of America

Movement for Every Body: An Inclusive Fitness Guide for Better Movement is sponsored and published by North Atlantic Books, an educational nonprofit based in the unceded Ohlone land Huichin (Berkeley, CA), that collaborates with partners to develop cross-cultural perspectives; nurture holistic views of art, science, the humanities, and healing; and seed personal and global transformation by publishing work on the relationship of body, spirit, and nature.

North Atlantic Books's publications are distributed to the US trade and internationally by Penguin Random House Publisher Services. For further information, visit our website at www.northatlanticbooks.com.

MEDICAL DISCLAIMER: The following information is intended for general information purposes only. Individuals should always see their health care provider before administering any suggestions made in this book. Any application of the material set forth in the following pages is at the reader's discretion and is their sole responsibility.

Library of Congress Cataloging-in-Publication Data
Names: Dernie, Marcia, author.
Title: Movement for every body : an inclusive fitness guide for better
   movement / Marcia Dernie, DPT.
Description: Berkeley, CA : North Atlantic Books, [2024] | Includes
   bibliographical references and index. | Summary: "An inclusive guide to
   improving mobility, building strength, and increasing flexibility for
   every body and any size, shape, and ability"– Provided by publisher.
Identifiers: LCCN 2023057133 (print) | LCCN 2023057134 (ebook) | ISBN
   9781623179960 (trade paperback) | ISBN 9781623179977 (ebook)
Subjects: LCSH: Movement education. | Physical fitness.
Classification: LCC GV452 .D47 2024 (print) | LCC GV452 (ebook) | DDC
   370.15/5–dc23/eng/20240105
LC record available at https://lccn.loc.gov/2023057133
LC ebook record available at https://lccn.loc.gov/2023057134

1 2 3 4 5 6 7 8 9 VERSA 29 28 27 26 25 24

North Atlantic Books is committed to the protection of our environment. We print on recycled paper whenever possible and partner with printers who strive to use environmentally responsible practices.

*To my mother, Marie Marcelle,
who always encouraged me to help
people in a million different ways,
and I never understood why. I finally
found my way, and I now understand.*

mèsi anpil manmi

Contents

Preface

Reading and Preparation Tips

We can't have *Movement for Every Body* without considering how to make the content in this book more accessible for every body to read. We all learn and process information in different ways that might vary from person to person depending on the content. This book is offered in text format (electronic or paper) and audio format. There are also accompanying videos for the movement activities included in each chapter.

If you have no idea where to begin, consider the following scenario: To learn a new recipe, would you rather read text instructions, listen to instructions, or watch a video? What do you need in order to be able to follow this recipe? Try to use your answers to these questions as a starting point for understanding your learning and processing needs. For example, when I'm learning a new recipe, I prefer text instructions with chunked sections I can read at my own pace while I make a checklist for grocery shopping. If I listen to instructions, I'll zone out after a few sentences. If I'm watching a video, I need closed captions with a faster playback speed and will often pause at many points. With this recipe example in mind, how would I apply these principles to reading this book? I might do better by reading the text and taking notes, unless I find better ways to stay engaged with audio. I would also speed up the video tutorials as I follow along in the text to absorb that information.

Ideas that may help with reading this book:

- Pace yourself while reading by setting timers or deciding the number of pages/sections to read at a time. Then take a break, and after that either read again if you want to, or stop.

- Make a reading schedule, and use a calendar to mark off days when you've read any pages or worked on the chapter activities.

- Talk about what you've read with a friend or aloud to yourself.

- For audio-based book reading, add an activity that makes reading physically engaging: take notes or use a fidget tool.

- For text-based book reading, add an activity that makes reading an auditory process: read out loud, or listen to music, white noise, or brown noise.

- For e-books, test out different fonts, page colors, and sizes. Some e-book applications have options for the Bionic Reading method or a dyslexia-specific font.

- For physical books, use a horizontal bookmark or ruler to keep your place on the page by sliding it downward as you read each line.

- Eliminate distractions by hydrating and nourishing before reading, and putting phones on Do Not Disturb if possible.

- Try reading in a place that makes you feel calm and peaceful, whether this is at home or elsewhere like a park.

- Consider creating a book club or reading along with a buddy to check in and have scheduled discussions.

Ideas that may help with watching the online videos:

- The videos can be accessed via phone, but consider using an iPad, computer screen, or smart TV for a bigger view.

- Remember that the playback speed is adjustable, which means the video can be slowed down or sped up to your preference.

- The video has an automated caption feature that will display spoken words on the screen.

- Check the video length before starting it, so you always know how long to expect to be watching it.

Preparation Tips

We all have different access to equipment and space, as well as different abilities and needs. This section provides items needed to complete the activities at the end of each chapter. The journaling activities can be completed in any position of comfort. The movement activities include positions that involve sitting, standing, and lying down on the floor. There are variations and ideas for modifications included with each specific activity, but it can be helpful to know before you get started what you may need in order to be successful.

Must Have

- Safe space to complete journaling and movement activities

- For journaling: notes app on phone, diary app, voice recorder, or paper journal

- For sitting exercises: sturdy, comfortable chair without wheels; couch; or bed

- For standing moves: clear area on floor, free of obstacles

- For floor exercises: blankets, pillows, towels for comfort

Nice to Have

- Small, hard items for support or alignment (yoga block, hardcover book, footstool)

- Large, tall, hard surface for balance (dining table, coffee table, entry table, wall, chair without wheels)

- Long handheld item for balance (broomstick, PVC pipe)

- Long, sturdy handheld item for positioning needs (yoga strap, flat sheet, belt)

- Soft items for comfort (pillows, bolsters, towels, blankets, yoga mat)

- Handheld weighted object (light dumbbell, light kettlebell, water bottle, ball)

- Camera with adequate storage for video feedback and measuring progress

- Large mirror for live feedback during movement

Introduction

I've always been a fairly active person. I spent my childhood playing kickball, climbing trees in my neighborhood, and playing sports in high school. During my time in high school and college, I bought into the prevalent fitness ideals that stated that women should be skinny, "cute," and small. I thought it was perfectly acceptable for only football players to use the weight room because women should only use the cardio equipment to get "toned." I disregarded years of shin splints, sprained ankles, torn shoulder muscles, and back pain because I believed that "pain is merely weakness leaving the body." I internalized these concepts as truths.

When I finally entered the weight room, the internalizations shifted, but they didn't improve. Instead, I developed an obsession with becoming the ideal strong and lean powerlifter. I was convinced that I had to be as small and shredded as possible to excel in powerlifting and to be respected in the sport. Thanks to my time in physical therapy school, I was embedded in a medical system rife with ableism and racism that fostered these body standards even more. During this time I worked out for about ten hours a week, did hot yoga, and did a lot of cardio while adhering to restrictive diets and binge-eating cycles. I kept up these routines, which shaped my movement and wellness practice, until I got sick.

My sickness started with stress. Adulting, toxic relationships, poor financial decisions, and unsustainable movement practices had finally caught up with me. I was burned out. The autoimmune illness that had been lurking in my immune system finally decided that now was the time to shine. Everything was fine until it wasn't. I was healthy and exercising normally until suddenly I wasn't. I reduced my daily exercise from three to four hours to barely fifteen minutes. I had terrible balance and was tripping over myself. Both my energy level and my executive functioning decreased. Everything quickly and abruptly declined. It all went downhill fast.

I'm confident that if I weren't a doctor of physical therapy, I would never have managed to climb back up that hill. I also realize that without internet communities like Disabled Girls Who Lift, I would not have been able to embrace my identity as a disabled person, my chronic illness, and my neurodivergent brain. And I am certain that without platforms like Decolonizing Fitness, Fitness 4 All Bodies, and Therapy for Black Girls, I could not have unpacked how much systems of oppression had affected my movement practice. These communities helped me to name what I was feeling, find terms for the systems I didn't agree with, and discover the power to take my autonomy back.

And that's what I hope this book does for you.

I took a long, hard look at my journey, including things that helped me along the way and experiences that bolstered me. I came to see that my journey is not unique, but understood that sharing it might benefit other people. Knowing what I've been through might help other people feel at home in their bodies after recent changes or injuries. It could help neurodivergent brains understand why they experience so much friction and frustration in fitness and medical systems that are built with one perspective in mind. Above all, my journey to wellness can help people who want to work out joyfully and safely without all the clickbait nonsense.

This book is for anyone who struggles with exercise, "health," fitness, or movement and feels disoriented, overwhelmed, or even ashamed. You may feel lost because the standard advice from shredded, fitbro white dudes is failing you. Or maybe you're overwhelmed because of the burdensome narratives telling you that you are broken and need to be fixed. Maybe you feel ashamed because the medical and fitness industry promotes codependency, unsustainable habits, and a wide range of contradictory, controversial opinions.

You're at the point in your movement journey where you're ready to toss aside the toxic nonsense and chase something real. You're ready to dig into discomfort and expand into something more. When you picked up this book, you had already made a choice to roll up your sleeves, reclaim your agency, and take control of your body. And I know that you will.

I see you through your struggle, and I know that you are done with feeling lost. And with every turn of the page, as this book holds your hand along this journey, you will find your way.

Will it be easy? No, of course not. Is it possible? Absolutely.

Appraise

appraise verb
ap·praise ə-ˈprāz
to evaluate the worth, significance, or status of

What Do We Need to Appraise?

When you assign value to your ability, your movement practices, and your expectations, the value you assign does not 100 percent come from you. More than likely a large portion came from the influences of toxic fitness culture and ableism, both of which are firmly rooted in the systems of oppression that stem from white supremacy. Now, you might be thinking: we're only a few sentences into the first chapter, and they're already pulling the race card! Hold your horses and put on your thinking cap. Consider this. The world as we know it was seized by colonizers and remolded to fit *their* ideal image. What is their ideal image? It's a person who's white (or pale-skinned), has straight hair, and is wealthy, thin, physically fit, and youthfully supple. This image is not only considered ideal but is also considered the superior image. According to Boston Medical Center, white supremacy is an institutionalized system of oppression of countries and people of color by white people in order to preserve their wealth, power, and privilege. Those who do not perfectly fit the philosophical or physical requirements of white supremacy often face barriers and discrimination. This is the root of the "-isms"—racism, sexism, ableism, and so on. This idealism also drives eugenics, which the National Human Genome Research Institute defines as a scientifically inaccurate theory that humans can be improved through selective breeding. Since the late 1800s, eugenicists and their practices have directly caused harm to marginalized populations via sterilization, segregation, and social exclusion aimed at "perfecting" human beings.

Our modern-day civilizations were born from an age where settlers deemed the lives of entire nations to be unworthy and cultures of entire peoples to be uncivilized. We cannot pretend that these actions, which stemmed from white supremacist ideals, have no bearing on every facet of our lives today, including how we view ability and movement. We must question ideals that work only for certain body types, backgrounds, and socioeconomic classes. And once we're done with that inquiry, we can truly step back and appraise our own thoughts and actions around movement and ability.

Toxic Fitness Culture and Standards

"Toxic fitness culture" is a term coined by Ilya Parker of Decolonizing Fitness. This cultural construct consists of two binary groups: one carrying exploited identities that mainstream fitness culture negatively impacts, and the other carrying traditionally accepted bodies that act as gatekeepers. How does this look in action? Here are a few examples:

- The marketing of fitness strictly for weight loss

- The use of shame and coercion to motivate people to work out

- Diet prescriptions from trainers who are not registered dietitians or nutritionists

- The belief that fitness has a body type and an aesthetic

- The belief that "experts" must exist in smaller bodies

- The belief that you aren't working hard if you haven't achieved thinness

- The belief that individual choices always lead to better health

It's not surprising that if we are surrounded by less-than-ideal standards for appearance and performance, we are also overwhelmed by exclusion from fitness spaces. Popular fitness and wellness influencers tend to be able-bodied, cisgendered, white or pale-skinned, straight-haired, skinny with noticeable abs, and of a certain socioeconomic class. And these same coaches and influencers believe that their aesthetics give them authority over the choices their clients should make about their own bodies. Fitness spaces welcome weight loss as the only goal and assume that anyone in a larger body wants to be smaller. Gyms employ coaches and trainers that fit a certain aesthetic, assuming everyone aspires to that ideal look or body type. Even our own algorithms have been programmed to feed us the same aesthetics. This is fatphobia in action. These coaches and influencers also belittle clients who choose to move differently, whether via mobility challenges like the "old man test," telling someone the exercise variation they chose is not hard enough, or labeling rest as laziness. These mainstream coaches and influencers also love to offer their diet plans as "helping people make better food choices for healthier lives." Not only is this fatphobia rearing its ugly head, but it also feeds into *healthism*—the idea that a person's health is completely determined by their individual actions.

We cannot assume that making all the "right" choices will lead to better health. Disability is an equal-opportunity employer. It doesn't care if you're a vegan with a "normal" body mass index (BMI), it doesn't care if you have visible abs, and it definitely doesn't care if you take no days off. Anyone can become chronically ill or mentally or physically disabled at any point in their lives. To claim otherwise is also naive. It is naive to think that individual choices can control all the variables that contribute to health. Social determinants of health (SDOH) alone create a wide array of health disparities and inequities. SDOH are environmental conditions that affect health, quality of life, and risk factors for health problems. SDOH are usually grouped into five domains: economic stability, education access, health care access, neighborhood, and community. For example, it doesn't matter if you diet hard and exercise harder if you live in a city like Flint, Michigan, that doesn't have access to clean water. And it would sound damn foolish to tell someone that daily exercise will prevent sickness if they work over forty hours a week and use crowded public transportation. Similarly, it would be ridiculous to tell a patient who traveled thirty miles to an appointment to eat "better" if there aren't any markets with fresh food in their neighborhood.

This feeling of exclusion also extends to medical and health care spaces. Health clinics ostracize a wide array of folks because medicine is also rooted in toxic fitness deals. Health care providers often assume that a fat person must lose weight to solve all their problems. At first glance, this idea seems scientific and real; but under a microscope, it doesn't hold up. For example, we know that all body types experience pain. So how can we tell someone with a higher BMI that losing weight will resolve their knee pain? This also applies to life-threatening illnesses. People in larger bodies often have whole-ass diseases and cancers that are missed because of this line of thinking. For example, we know that anyone with lungs can experience respiratory issues, but for some reason "morbidly" obese patients have delayed diagnosis and care for pulmonary embolism (a blood clot in the lungs). And before you ask, "morbidly" is in quotation marks because using BMI as the determining factor of health is pure foolishness. The BMI formula was created by a mathematician who based it on a sample of white men. Since the formula (weight divided by squared height) doesn't distinguish tissue type or distribution, it unsurprisingly fails populations outside of that sample. Medical doctors will also provide wordy diet handouts recommending healthier choices without ever asking if their patient has access to a grocery store. These diets often display a Eurocentric bias by labeling cultural foods as unhealthy choices. Absolutely none of this is acceptable.

Toxic fitness culture wants us to believe in the "no pain, no gain" motto and to sweat-shame ourselves into thinness to achieve healthy, fit bodies. This narrative persists because it is profitable. It is profitable for us to constantly strive for perfection, to despise our physical appearance, and to hire "experts" to make us feel inferior. The corporations that sell us lightening creams and diet meal plans do not care about our health; they care about their profits. The gyms and fitness spaces that sell shame and weight loss do not care about our well-being; they care about their bottom line. This connects back to white supremacy, which is permeated with settler ideologies and includes oppressive mechanisms at every turn. The narrative is that our bodies are inferior unless we are the right color, a particular size, and have a certain level of physical ability. The bad news is that this is no coincidence. The good news is that we have the ability to unsubscribe from these deliberately destructive messages.

Ableism and Disability Identity

Ableism, as defined by the Center for Disability Rights, is when people with disabilities are devalued or discriminated against. Ableism often rests on the assumption that disabled people are broken and need to be fixed. How does this look in action? Here are a few examples:

- Applauding a disabled person for doing something ordinary like going to the gym; i.e., viewing them as inspiration porn
- Believing a disabled person is incapable of engaging in everyday activities like working, voting, driving, or parenting
- The belief that a disabled person can't be attractive or participate in athletics
- The belief that needing or prioritizing rest is lazy
- The belief that using exercise modifications or taking more rest breaks is less than
- The belief that exercises must have a certain intensity or take a certain length of time to be effective

You might feel shame for not being able to perform a "full" yoga pose or guilt for being the only person in a group fitness class to take breaks or modify exercises. That is the voice of internalized ableism. You could experience grief and sadness over the physical abilities you once possessed before your injury, illness, or disability "held you back." You might even feel helpless and wonder if you will ever enjoy movement or exercise. Which is totally normal!

But guess what? The beauty of our diversity is that different bodies can move in various ways. Different bodies have different abilities, and that's perfectly okay. Disabled and chronically ill folks are most certainly capable of finding movement that works for whatever body shows up that day. Having a disability does require lots of acceptance, mindfulness, and self-advocacy, and lots of accommodations. It does not require feeling shame about one's situation or navigating a society that was created eugenically for the able-bodied. It does require us to remember that less ability does not equal less worth. It's also worth mentioning that we cannot feed into the idea that every single disability needs curing, fixing, or mending. And we've got to stop buying into the cycle of learned helplessness, the idea that our lives and situations are unchangeable and that we must submit.

You might also be wondering whether some of these labels—disabled, chronically ill—apply to you. And for the people in the back, a disability is any condition that makes it more difficult to perform certain activities or interact with the world. These activity limitations and participation restrictions can be caused by physical or mental issues, invisible or visible conditions, or a combination of them all. A physical disability may include a condition that is visible, such as cerebral palsy, spinal cord injury, or limb differences. A physical disability can also include conditions that are not visible, such as blindness, deafness, autoimmune disorders, epilepsy, or postural orthostatic tachycardia syndrome (POTS). Both types of disabilities affect the ability to perform activities and interact with the world in a physical way. For example:

- A gym goer with cerebral palsy may have difficulty holding a dumbbell.

- A wheelchair user with a spinal cord injury may have difficulty accessing gym equipment.

- A deaf athlete may have issues following along during virtual exercise classes.

- Someone with POTS might pass out in a heated yoga class or a warm fitness room.

Bear in mind that dichotomous thinking is not being encouraged here. A person can have multiple physical disabilities, multiple invisible and visible conditions, as well as mental disabilities. There are many overlaps between physical and mental disabilities. Some physical disabilities cause mental disabilities, and some mental disabilities cause physical manifestations. A mental disability will usually include conditions that are not visible, such as anxiety, depression, personality disorders, posttraumatic stress disorder (PTSD), dementia, or diagnoses that cause executive dysfunction and sensory processing issues such as autism, attention-deficit/hyperactivity disorder (ADHD), or diseases involving the brain. It's important to note that trauma, dysfunction in childhood, and stressful events can lead to or exacerbate existing emotional dysregulation and executive dysfunction. These mental disabilities affect a person's ability to perform activities and interact with the world in material ways. For instance:

- An autistic person may have issues in a loud gym with blaring lights.

- Someone with anxiety may avoid hiring a coach if the process involves extra steps to get more information.

- A person with trauma may have a somatic response to a gym partner who, intentionally or unintentionally, says their trigger words.

- A person with brain fog from an autoimmune condition might drop out of group fitness classes after being unable to keep up.

Each person's journey with disability is unique, and there are many ways to embark upon this adventure of self-exploration. First, I encourage you to explore the depth of the language within the disability community. For example, do any of the terms "disabled," "wheelchair user," "spoonie," "crip," "chronic illness," or "neurodivergent" resonate with you? Understand that *disabled* is not a bad word, but if you choose to identify with other terms, that is okay too. What is not okay is someone else correcting the language you choose to describe yourself.

Spoonie is derived from "The Spoon Theory," an article by Christine Miserandino, where the author uses a limited number of daily "spoons" as a symbol to represent the limited units of energy available to complete tasks with daily variable energy requirements. Many people with chronic illnesses and mental health conditions talk about "how many spoons" they have left or "being out of spoons" because it's a great metaphor to describe how needs and abilities can vary from day to day for people who have dynamic disabilities. Meanwhile, *crip* is a reappropriated term from "cripple," a weaponized word used with the intent to harm. *Crip* is not universally accepted by every disabled person, as is the case with any of the terms that have been sprinkled in here. *Chronic illness* is used to describe unseen or invisible health issues that will never go away. This term is not usually used for physical disabilities. *Neurodivergent* is used to describe folks who process information in a way that is different from the norm, i.e., different from those who are "neurotypical." Whether neurodivergence is paired with a formal diagnosis may depend on the individual and their circumstances, as neurodivergence can encompass conditions such as autism, ADHD, PTSD, bipolar disorder, and traumatic brain injury.

Second, explore whether person-first language or identity-first language resonates most with you. With person-first language, humanity is placed in the forefront. You would call yourself a person with a disability or a person with a chronic illness. With identity-first language, a holistic view is preferred, so you would call yourself a disabled person or a chronically ill person. Many communities default to identity-first language, while others do not seem to have a standard. Some communities love euphemisms such as *fighter, warrior,* and *survivor,* while others abhor them. There is no right or wrong when it comes to your personal preference for language that describes you. Dive into your specific community or experience and see what feels right for you. Keep in mind that each experience is different, and you may find spaces that do not feel inclusive, safe, or intersectional. A disabled space might not be free of racism, transphobia, fatphobia, and so on.

How does a person with a disability find community? It usually starts with the diagnosis. Obtaining a formal diagnosis in the American health care system is neither simple nor cheap. There are many diagnoses with specific criteria that pose barriers to getting a diagnosis thanks to the cost of diagnostic procedures, access to diagnostic facilities, and insurance coverage, because the health care system in the United States is restrictive by design and is rooted in white supremacy. There are also situations where a formal diagnosis helps one person get accommodations at work or school, but the same diagnosis makes no difference for another person. Particularly when it comes to neurodivergence stemming from autism and/or ADHD, many are choosing to forgo formal diagnosis and opt for self-diagnosis. If you find the second option is worth digging into, Dr. Megan Anna Neff offers self-assessment and coping resources on their website NeurodivergentInsights.com. With a diagnosis or a name for your condition, you can find support through organizations specific to that condition and get involved with that community. You could also browse Reddit, Twitter, or online communities like Inspire (www.inspire.com) or Stuff That Works (www.stuffthatworks.health) to find folks with similar diagnoses, conditions, and/or symptoms.

Here are some popular hashtags that appear on several social media platforms that can help you find your community (and there are plenty of others that aren't listed below):

- #ActuallyAutistic

- #DisabilityTwitter

- #AuDHD

- #NEISvoid

- #MigraineChat

- #LupusChat

- #hEDS

- #ChronicallyIll

- #DisabledBlackLivesMatter

- #DisabilityPrideMonth

- #DisabilityPride

Journaling Activity: Appraise and Reframe

Hopefully at this point we've steered ourselves in the direction of defining our own standards when it comes to mobility, ability, fitness, and health. We've assessed what the world has fed our brains to believe, and now it's time to assess what we want to believe. Changing a belief or behavior is no small task. It takes effort to explore the shadows and bring darker thoughts to light. And this effort must be consistent over time. We also have to remember to lead this continual exploration with self-compassion. Understand that you are worth the time and the space. You won't leap over every hurdle on the first run, and that's okay. It won't be easy to process thoughts and feelings that make us uncomfortable; expecting otherwise would be foolish.

Setting yourself up for success with movement starts with moving your thoughts. If your thoughts around mobility and health are fed by guilt, shame, or fear, your movement practice will be sabotaged before it's even started. By becoming more aware of our thoughts, we can interrupt this vicious cycle. Let's start with deprogramming negative thoughts about movement and uploading better ones. Set aside time for this activity, and feel free to return to it whenever a negative thought pops up. If it's helpful for you, set a timer to complete the activity after reading the instructions.

What you will need for this activity:

- Paper and pen or note-taking phone app

- Peaceful and comfortable space

- Five to ten minutes of dedicated time

INSTRUCTIONS

1. Write down a negative thought you've had about movement.

2. Consider how toxic fitness culture or ableism whispered that idea into your brain.

3. Explore whether this thought takes internal or external causes into consideration.

4. Explore whether the experience or thought is a forever thing or a temporary situation.

5. Explore whether it is a global issue or specific to one environment.

6. Write down a reframed version of this thought.

I'll give you a few examples, along with the thought process that could lead to the reframe.

- I get hurt every time I lift heavy. I'll never get a deadlift PR [personal record]!

  - Who decides when I should PR my deadlift? Am I any less for taking longer than other people?

  - What happens when I do get hurt? Is it really every single time? Have I even tried anything different?

  - Do I only get hurt when lifting heavy? Do I notice when my body is in pain or needs rest? What have I been doing right after I do get hurt?

  - *New thought:* I didn't get enough mobility/water/rest/recovery work the last time I was training heavy. All the other times I trained heavy, I didn't get hurt. I can also be proactive and work on more mobility stuff so I can handle more load.

- I can't do any of these mobility challenges, and I'm only in my thirties!

  - Who says my body has to be able to move in a certain way? Do I need to listen to social media influencers tell me what's right for the body I live in?

- I only recently started practicing these mobility challenges, so it makes sense that they're difficult for me. When I watch videos, I'm looking at people with different abilities who have been practicing for a much longer time.

- Does this mobility challenge even apply to my life? Does it matter if I can stand on one leg and put on a shoe?

- *New thought:* I know my ability is defined by me, and I'm not worth any less if I can't move the way someone else does.

I hate going to the gym. I'll never get into exercise.

- Is there a reason I hate going to the gym? Is it the people I go with? The people I see there? Do I wear gym clothes that make me uncomfortable? Is the gym too loud and bright and overwhelming? Am I unhappy with the time it takes to prepare for a gym workout and travel there and back?

- Was there ever a time when I did enjoy exercise? What did that look like? Where was that? Who was I with?

- *New thought:* I don't like the gym because it doesn't feel like a safe space, and I need to feel like I'm free from judgment to enjoy fitness and movement.

I'm too old to start doing yoga poses.

- Why do I feel there is an age limit to this activity? Is it because all the influencers and the people in the yoga photos are youthful and visibly fit? Is it because society says I must like low-impact group classes and nothing else?

- Who have I talked to about my desire to start doing yoga poses? Who do I follow online that looks or moves like me? How can I better support myself and see this through?

- *New thought:* I feel out of place trying to exercise in a group with young people, and I don't know where to start. I'm going to find people like me and learn more with them.

- My chronic illness is worse. I can't do anything, and I'm gaining weight.

  - Where can I fit more space for rest and ease in my life, to free up energy for movement? Who can I ask to help me with everyday tasks to free up time?

  - How can I change my idea of what I used to be able to do and break it down into something small that I might be able to do now? What type of environment would be helpful for me to enjoy movement? If I can only do ten minutes instead of the sixty minutes I did before, is that better than nothing?

  - Do I need to get professional help to figure out how to safely move again? Do I follow anyone with a chronic illness who does my preferred exercises? Am I willing to try something new?

  - *New thought:* I feel sad that I can't move the way I used to, but not hopeless. It will take some work and exploration to still enjoy movement, because it will have to be in a different way.

Movement Activity: Connect to the Breath

The first step in the self-appraisal process was to become aware of the thoughts in our minds. The next step in the process is connection to our bodies. We can build that mind-body connection by starting with the yogic practice called *pranayama*. *Pranayama* is the yogic practice of focusing on the breath, which brings awareness of and control over body and mind. Yoga is an organized philosophical system with many parts, organized into eight limbs: *yama, niyama, asana, pranayama, pratyahara, dharana, dhyana,* and *samadhi.* In this book we will directly explore yoga's physical and breathing practices (*asana* and *pranayama*) and indirectly touch on the others along the way.

Taking the time to pause and reflect on our breath with intentional practice has many benefits:

- It allows us to examine our current mood.

- It gives us space to explore our thoughts.

- It gives us space to explore our bodily feelings.

- It allows us to work toward a target bodily feeling.

- It strengthens our control of breath during rest and stress.

The main mover of breathwork is the diaphragm muscle, which sits at the base of the chest. In a perfect world, when you breathe in, the diaphragm contracts and creates space for the lungs to take in air. When you breathe out, the diaphragm relaxes into place as the lungs empty. Other muscles help to move the ribs around, which is totally fine. But sometimes if the diaphragm isn't doing its job, these accessory muscles try to pick up the slack. For some of us this is due to nerve injuries or structural problems; for others it's lack of awareness and connection. Dedicating a focused effort to using that main mover for breathwork will allow you to have a more efficient breathing pattern, in addition to the mood and physiological benefits. It's also worth noting that if you don't have a handle on using your diaphragm at rest, you definitely won't have a handle on it during stress. This can mean that once you get flustered at work and your heart starts racing, you can't calm down, or it could mean you can't catch your breath during a workout. For many, diaphragmatic breathing requires some practice because it can be tough to create new movement patterns. In the beginning, try tactile cues—like placing a hand on your chest, or lying down and placing a book on your belly—to help you learn. Explore visual cues like looking in a mirror, using a front-facing mobile camera, or reviewing a self-recording to gain more body awareness.

What you will need for this activity:

- Paper and pen or note-taking phone app

- Peaceful and comfortable space

- Ten to fifteen minutes of dedicated time

- Optional mirror or phone to record for feedback

INSTRUCTIONS

1. Stand, lie down, or sit comfortably in any position.

2. If you're able to, place one arm on your chest and the other on your belly.

3. Try five to ten cycles of each breathing exercise described below. You can take breaks between each exercise for as long as you need to.

4. Take notes on how each breathing exercise made you feel.

5. Plan for the situations in which you can use each breathing exercise.

You can visit my website at www.MovementforEveryBody.org to find videos that accompany these instructions.

Belly Breath

Belly Breath, or diaphragmatic breathing, is the "perfect" breathing pattern as described earlier. This breath can be practiced at rest and may eventually become your default pattern. For this breath we will be breathing through the nose. If this is uncomfortable, breathe through the mouth instead.

1. Assume a comfortable position.

   ▪ If lying down, place a book or your hand on your belly.

   ▪ If seated, place one hand on your chest and the other on your belly.

   ▪ If standing, make sure your feet are even and your weight is balanced.

2. Take a big breath in. As you inhale, imagine that your belly is a balloon filling with air.

3. Let the big breath out. As you exhale, imagine your balloon is rapidly losing air.

4. If that went well, consider adding "box breathing" to this Belly Breath, as described in the next two steps:

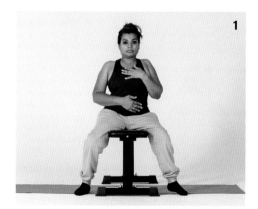
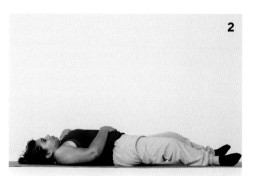

5. Take a big breath in as you count to three, and then hold your breath for three seconds.

6. Let the big breath out as you count to three, and then hold that empty belly for three seconds.

Possible uses for Belly Breath plus box breathing:

■ Practice during daily ordinary activities

■ Practice alongside daily exercises

■ Use during a moment of unexpected panic

■ Take calm breaths while going to sleep

■ Take calm breaths while journaling

Lion's Breath

Lion's Breath is a calming and cooling breath. This breath can help expel heat and pent-up energy. For this breath we will be breathing in through the nose and out through the mouth.

1. Assume a comfortable position.

   ■ If lying down, place a book or your hand on your belly.

   ■ If seated, place one hand on your chest and the other on your belly.

   ■ If standing, make sure your feet are even and your weight is balanced.

2. Take a big breath in through the nose and fill your belly with air.

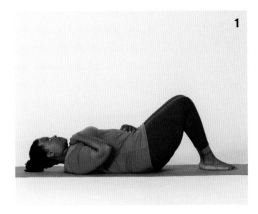
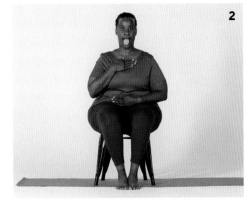

3. Open your mouth and stick out your tongue as far as is comfortable, and let the big breath out through the mouth. As you exhale, make a "haaaaaa" sound.

Possible uses for Lion's Breath:

- Use after a moment of heavy exertion

- Use between activities when you can't seem to catch your breath

- Use during a stressful moment when your heart is racing

Bunny Breath

Bunny Breath is a sniffing breath pattern that can help us center ourselves. For this breath we will be breathing through the nose. If this is uncomfortable, skip it entirely. Do not force it.

1. Assume a comfortable position.

   - If lying down, place a book or your hand on your belly.

   - If seated, place one hand on your chest and the other on your belly.

   - If standing, make sure your feet are even and your weight is balanced.

2. Take multiple sniffs in through your nose until your belly is completely filled with air.

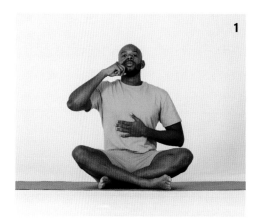 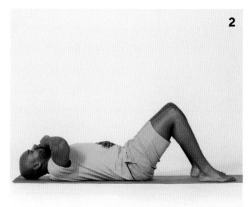

3. Let out one long exhale through your nose until your belly is completely emptied.

Possible uses for Bunny Breath:

■ Use during a moment of unexpected panic

■ Use between activities when you can't seem to center your thoughts

■ Use during a stressful moment when your heart is racing

Ocean Breath

Ocean Breath or Ujayi Breath is a focusing breath that can help direct your energy and focus on the task or thought at hand. The aim is to keep this breath at a constant pace and consistently *loud*. We will be breathing through the nose with the lips sealed. If this is uncomfortable, breathe through the mouth instead.

1. Assume a comfortable position.

■ If lying down, place a book or your hand on your belly.

■ If seated, place one hand on your chest and the other on your belly.

■ If standing, make sure your feet are even and your weight is balanced.

2. Take a big breath in through the nose, and fill your belly with air.

3. Open your mouth to let out the big breath. Pretend you are fogging a mirror.

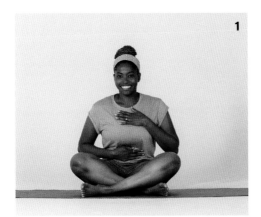
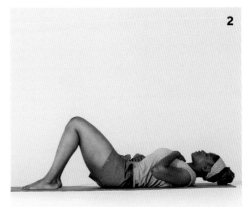

4. Take a big breath in through the nose, and fill your belly with air.

5. Keep your lips sealed, and let out the big breath as if you are fogging a mirror.

6. Repeat steps 4 and 5.

Possible uses for Ocean Breath:

■ Get steady while holding an exercise position

■ Center before a big lift or during a long run

■ Practice during daily ordinary activities

■ Practice alongside daily exercises

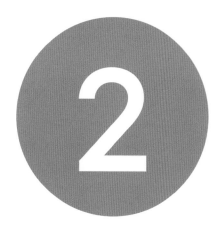

Assess

assess verb
as·sess ə-ˈses
to determine the rate or amount of

What Do We Need to Assess?

We can become more aware of our movement patterns through self-study and assessment. As we examine our movement patterns and body motions, we assess them without shame or judgment. We don't assign value to areas that are supposedly limited, and we don't feel guilty about muscle groups that are weak. We evaluate and investigate to better understand our bodies, not to belittle them. Once we become aware of our movement patterns and adopt a shame-free mindset, we inch closer to actually enjoying movement. (If shameful thoughts pop back up, pause and reflect on the journaling activity from chapter 1 to get you through that moment.) In addition to studying our movement patterns and assessing how our joints move, we will also explore how our bodies work and what routines we can employ to improve our nervous system regulation, sleep, and nourishment.

The self-assessment of our routines and how our bodies actually move may require input from a trained professional on your care team. You may want to pass this book along to your trusted provider for the go-ahead if you have undergone surgery, experienced significant changes in your physical or mental health, or have current medical implants. If that doesn't apply right now, keep it in mind when you return to this book in the future, because bodies can change over time.

What Moves Us?

Your self-assessment does not require an in-depth knowledge of anatomy, but a brief overview and introduction of a few terms may prove useful. Don't worry; it won't get too technical or wordy! But a little background might help you understand the magic of our bodies, which are full of processes that function without us even thinking about it. To aid comprehension, we group these functions into "systems." In reality, all the systems influence each other and work in tandem. A list of our bodily systems is provided below; in this book we'll focus briefly on the first two.

Body Systems

- Nervous system: brain, spinal cord, and nerves that communicate and control body functions

- Musculoskeletal system: muscle, bones, and soft tissues that provide structure and move both body parts and substances

- Vestibular system: structures and fluid within the inner ear that work to coordinate eye movements and orient the body in space; a part of the nervous system

- Cardiopulmonary system: heart and lungs, which provide oxygen and nutrients throughout the body via the blood and its vessels (which are also part of the system)

- Urinary (renal) system: kidney, ureters, bladder, and urethra, which all work together to filter out waste from the blood

- Digestive system: mouth, esophagus, stomach, intestines, liver, and rectum, which all work together to break down food for nutrient absorption

- Skin (integumentary) system: skin, hair, nails, and glands, which work to receive information and serve as an outer protective layer

- Endocrine system: glands (hypothalamus, pituitary, thyroid, adrenal, pancreas, and gonads) that regulate biological processes by secreting hormones through ducts

- Exocrine system: exocrine glands (located in mouth, chest, pancreas, skin, and small intestine) that secrete substances (sweat, mucus, oil, and milk) to help organs function

- Reproductive system: either vagina, uterus, fallopian tubes, and ovaries, which produce eggs (ova); or penis, testicles, epididymis, vas deferens, and prostate gland, which produces sperm

- Immune system: a system of cells, organs, and vessels that fight disease-causing germs and changes within the body

- Lymphatic system: a network of tissues and vessels that circulate lymph fluid back into the blood; a part of the immune system

Nervous System

The nervous system is made up of the brain, spinal cord, and nerves. The brain and spinal cord make up the central nervous system. The nerves make up the peripheral nervous system, which is further split into the autonomic nervous system and the somatic system. All involuntary muscular movements, including breathing, heart rate, digestion, sweating, sneezing, and coughing, are controlled by the autonomic nervous system. The autonomic nervous system, in turn, is made up of the parasympathetic nervous system and the sympathetic nervous system. The parasympathetic side focuses on involuntary actions for resting and digesting, while the sympathetic side is all about fight or flight. Although the somatic system controls all voluntary muscle actions, we can use voluntary actions to influence involuntary pathways (more on that later).

The nervous system will always try to learn and adapt in response to change. Our nerves demonstrate *neuroplasticity,* or the ability to regenerate, restructure, or adapt to change. The kinds of changes our nerves can respond to include moving from a warm environment to a cold one, wearing a new pair of shoes, trying a new exercise at a new gym, or sustaining a physical injury. In response to change, our nervous system can create either shortcuts (good) or compensations (not always good). For example, if you drive to the same place every day at the same time, do you ever feel like you got there without thinking about it? That's your nervous system creating a shortcut, which is usually good—unless you were supposed to drive somewhere else! On the other hand, if you've ever sprained an ankle, do you ever notice that even after it heals you put more weight on the "good" side? That's your nervous system creating a compensation, which was helpful in the beginning but not so much once you've healed up.

Our nervous system receives information through our five senses and our body position, and that information is used by both our voluntary and involuntary pathways. Once we've processed that information, our nervous system sends signals to our body and tells it what to do. Let's say we're about to do a push-up on top of a workout bench. Our bodies automatically contract postural muscles to keep us upright once we see the bench. We urge ourselves to fire up our arms and take a breath as soon as we touch the bench. The angle at which our elbows are positioned tells our bodies which muscles to engage in order to raise us back up. Our bodies unconsciously raise our heart rates to pump more blood as our muscles contract. Many of us go through this process in the blink of an eye, but people with neurological disorders might not. Neurological problems can also cause "faulty" messages to be transmitted from the brain to the muscles. For example, in this case, the timing of elbow locking may be off, a hand tremor may make it hard to stay on the bench, or the heart rate may remain elevated even after movement has stopped. Neurological disorders can also lead to "faulty" messages at default, causing muscles to overfire (hypertonicity) or underfire (hypotonicity) before movement even happens.

TL;DR: NERVOUS SYSTEM

- Messages received from our senses and receptors are sent to the brain.

- The brain sends messages to our body for both involuntary and voluntary actions.

- Paying attention to our bodies can alter automatic involuntary actions (e.g., breathing).

- The nervous system adapts in response to change, but not always in a good way.

- "Faulty" messages can lead to muscle spasms or twitches, body tremors, or flaccidity (low muscle tone or hypotonicity).

Musculoskeletal System

The musculoskeletal system is made up of muscle tissues, connective tissues, and bones. The body has three types of muscle tissue: visceral (often known as smooth), cardiac, and skeletal. Skeletal movement is voluntary, but visceral and heart movement are not. For example, to read these words you may have to hold a book in your hands and coordinate balancing the book as you turn the pages; but you don't have to focus on squeezing your heart to pump blood or moving food through your system when taking a snack break while reading. The muscles in the body are connected to the bones by connective tissue. Ligaments join bone to bone, while tendons connect muscles to bones. Tendons can contract, while ligaments cannot. Other connective tissues—including the meniscus in the knees, the labrum in the hips and shoulders, and bursae sacs in most joints—cushion our joints to support movement and protect against injury.

Bones, tissue, and muscles seem like they should function in a straightforward way. Our muscles are made to flow in specific directions, and the joints move in specific ways. But it is not that simple. The musculoskeletal system is all interconnected, so a problem at one joint can cause a problem at others. For example, how the foot moves can affect how the knee moves, which can result in hip pain. On top of that, all the body's systems are interconnected, so illnesses or issues in other body systems may also lead to musculoskeletal issues. Here are a few examples of how that could work:

- After knee surgery, a person could have trouble engaging muscles in the affected leg and bending that knee because of inflammation.

- A person with chronic obstructive pulmonary disorder may have a rib cage shaped differently from that of a person without lung problems.

- Someone with multiple sclerosis might trip over their own feet because they can't feel where their feet are without looking at them.

- An albino person might have chronic neck pain because they tilt their head to accommodate vision issues.

- A person with endometriosis might have tight hips and a stiff spine from constantly being in a fetal position due to pain.

- Someone with carpal tunnel syndrome might drop objects or have trouble opening jars because of nerve pain and faulty signals.

- A person with Ehlers-Danlos syndrome has hypermobile, unstable joints because of loose connective tissue, while a person with ankylosing spondylitis has hypomobile, stiff joints because of inflammation.

- Someone with impaired vision could have issues with balance, regardless of whether their joints are stable and sturdy.

- A person who has experienced physical trauma may overtrain and injure themselves more often, regardless of ability, because they're disconnected from their body.

Does Mental Health Matter?

We need to look at how each component of our bodies moves and at how the brain influences this movement. We cannot disconnect the physical from the mental. We already know that physical disabilities can lead to mental disabilities, and mental disabilities can result in physical manifestations. It's also crucial to know that emotional state can affect physical health and performance negatively, with or without having a mental illness or disability. Daily events and stressors can affect task performance by messing with our brains and bodies. Trying to engage in movement without recognizing the mess only creates a bigger one. For example, have you ever had a long, stressful day at work and then find yourself extra clumsy in the weight room? Have you ever been so overcome by a sad event that you struggle to get started with your daily walk?

Once we are aware of our mental state, we can adapt and adjust our movements to better suit that moment's needs. We can self-regulate our mental headspace and behaviors by choosing movements that support rather than aggravate our arousal levels. We can also self-regulate our physiological state, or the condition of the body and its functions, by finding our "window of tolerance." Finding this optimal zone of arousal (or alertness) allows us to function more effectively, with a normalized physiological state. The bad news is that dysregulation is often involuntary. Arousal levels can get out of whack from sensory processing disorders, trauma responses, everyday stressors, or demanding events. The good news is that we can sometimes voluntarily bring ourselves back to that window of tolerance by pausing in the moment. This may be a hard ask for those who have permanent injuries or congenital neuromuscular disorders, or who have experienced past trauma, as the disconnect between body and mind can be greater in those circumstances. When it comes to asking for outside help, often the licensed practitioners who can assist would be psychotherapists, occupational therapists, and sometimes physical therapists (especially those who work with neurological conditions or disabled kiddos). Let's explore what a state of hyperarousal or hypoarousal can look like for some folks, along with techniques that might help. And, huge disclaimer: there is no one-size-fits-all approach for emotional and sensory regulation techniques.

HYPERAROUSED STATE	HYPOAROUSED STATE
▪ Fight, flight, fawn (sympathetic state)	▪ Freeze or faint (sympathetic state), rest (parasympathetic state)
▪ Feelings of agitation and overwhelm	▪ Feelings of sluggishness or numbness
▪ Increased heart and breath rate	▪ Decreased body awareness
▪ Increased muscle tension or spasms	▪ Decreased muscle tension
▪ Inability to sit still or slow down	▪ Inability to get started or wake up
▪ Desire for stimulating environment	▪ Desire for quiet environment

CALMING, GROUNDING TECHNIQUES FOR HYPERAROUSAL	INVIGORATING, GROUNDING TECHNIQUES FOR HYPOAROUSAL
▪ Heavy exertion to "push" out the energy; or gentle movement to bring down the heart rate	▪ Gentle movement to slowly stimulate blood flow; or high-energy movements to bring up the heart rate
▪ Introduce rocking, swinging, or vibration	▪ Introduce tapping, squeezing, or vibration
▪ Practice Lion's Breath to cool down and focus	▪ Practice Ocean Breath to build heat and focus
▪ Remove bright lights and loud sounds	▪ Add light and rhythmic sounds

What Else Matters?

All things in life require exploration for growth. Movement is no exception. This book has some great words and ideas, but it will be your work and active exploration that make a difference. This active exploration also requires a sense of connection to ourselves as we float around in the real world. We've learned how our bodies and brains function, but we will have to work to remain consciously aware of these processes on a daily basis, ranging from everyday moments to stressful work days to cumbersome personal events. The way we nourish our bodies with sleep, food, and hydration matters in all those moments.

Getting Better Rest

We all need restful . . . rest. This is where the magic happens for our bodies. We can start by exploring parts of our day where rest can be better prioritized, whether it's stepping away from your desk at lunch or taking a silly little walk for your mental health. We can also dive into our sleep habits. Sleep is important! There are many variables within our control that can contribute to better sleep. Exploring the variables and creating better sleep hygiene can make all the difference. It is quite natural if hearing these "simple" suggestions elicits an instant eye roll. We all know there's a fine line between cringe and helpfulness. Try to approach these recommendations with curiosity rather than skepticism. I don't have your solutions; only you do. These suggestions are ideas to spark your personal journey, not concrete solutions. It is also worth noting the amount of privilege required to even consider taking these steps to improve your sleep. Seeing an allergist or getting a sleep study would be hard without health insurance or affordable access to care. Dissecting old habits and forming new ones can be overwhelming without access to a support network, which may include hired help like therapists, physicians, and coaches. Improving sleep habits would also be impossible without housing security and a safe place to lay your head.

Here are are some general tricks for better sleep hygiene—take what works, and leave what doesn't:

- Create a set sleep schedule based on your needs and a routine based on the time of day when you function best.

- Replace old mattresses and pillows when you can.

- Use extra pillows to support your preferred sleeping positions.

- Explore whether fitness-tracking straps, watches, or apps can help you learn more about sleep quality and daily energy expenditures.

- To investigate causes of snoring, check for allergies or sleep apnea.

- Try journaling, gentle movement, or *pranayama* before bed to calm the mind.

- Try mouth guards for teeth grinding, and consider consulting a dentist for custom options.

- Try cutting off usage of electronics at a certain time, storing them away from the bed, or using built-in electronic features like night mode and screen timers.

- Try sleeping on a wedge pillow or elevating your mattress to relieve reflux issues. If you need medications, find a good GI (gastroenterologist).

- See if making a custom YouTube or Spotify playlist for music, white noise, or background sounds is helpful.

- See if music, eye masks, ear plugs, aromatherapy, or weighted blankets help you stay asleep at night. (If nothing over the counter works, get a sleep study if you have access to care.)

- Consult with your providers and movement professionals to manage pain, or try different types of movement before bed.

- Consult with your mental health providers to create healthy coping mechanisms and self-care strategies.

- Consult with your health care providers to review new medications or side effects of existing meds.

Tackle one thing at a time. Realize that this takes time, and effort, and sometimes money. For example, I used to wake up feeling like I had just finished eating a pizza and then someone tossed me into quicksand. Mornings are still the worst part of my day painwise, but after tons of trial and error, seeking out safe providers, and a few years (yes, years!), on a perfect day I sleep well. I have the absolute silence, darkness, and stillness I need thanks to my weighted blanket, earplugs, and eye masks. Thanks to my wedge pillow and my reflux medications, my stomach acids stay where they're supposed to stay as I sleep. Thanks to a countertop full of moisturizers, my throat, nose, and eyes are prevented from crusting up at night. Shout-out to my allergist, who helped me identify my triggers so I can stop being a mouth breather. Much love to my alarm clock, which helps me keep the bedroom phone free. And thank goodness for the bulleted list taped to my closet door, which helps me remember all the steps in my sleep routine.

Also note that your journey is yours. Try not to emulate your partner's or loved one's habits or copy someone's routine from social media. Play around with one variable at a time, and create your own restful rituals and sleep hygiene. For example, the times when I take lunch, exercise, and go to sleep were different from my those of my partner and siblings. My friends don't use any of the sleep aids I mentioned and don't need to see a GI, allergist, and neurologist to get better sleep. What works for everybody else to rest well does not work for me, and vice versa.

Getting Better Nourishment

We all need nourishment and hydration to thrive, because our bodies need energy to spend energy. Getting proper nourishment can be hard if we're dealing with health problems, budget issues, family members with different diets, and other barriers. Feeding ourselves and drinking enough can also be tough when we're contending with toxic fitness and diet cultures. I would encourage you to assess current eating habits without judgment, but with curiosity.

Here are some quick tips and tricks for better nourishment:

- Don't sit down at your desk or on the couch without a glass of water.

- Don't leave your house without an emotional support water jug or bottle.

- Set timers and alarms if you forget to eat at regular intervals or struggle with hunger cues.

- If it's helpful, include mealtimes and snacks on your calendar or to-do lists.

- Think about how you can add an extra fruit or veggie to meals that don't have them.

- Consult with an allergist, registered dietitian, or GI if you can't find safe foods.

- Seek the care of mental health providers to work through big emotions around food and diet.

- Explore food delivery services, curbside service, or bulk shopping to cut down on food shopping burdens.

- Explore frozen foods, prechopped foods, and prepared items to cut down on food prep burdens.

- Play around with food prepping by cooking bulk meals or having certain items always available, to cut down on cooking burdens.

- Explore whether you enjoy eating the same meals or a variety on a day-to-day basis, to cut down on food waste.

- Figure out the best ways to store and pack your foods for easy access and to cut down on food waste.

Journaling Activity: Creating More Space

Going full throttle into self-exploration and movement is a whole-ass project that will require consistent effort and practice. With that in mind, we need to be sure we're taking care of ourselves with frequent mental check-ins and assessments of our daily routines. We cannot be in tune with movement if we're not in tune with our emotional states and surrounding environment. Let's set the solid foundation of building emotional regulation skills and making solid routines by making a couple of lists. List making can also be a form of journaling, especially helpful for folks who are fans of bullet points and quick phrases *(me!)*. This practice might even lead to setting new boundaries with yourself and others. Please note: you are welcome to break up this activity over multiple sessions. It does not have to be done all at once!

What you will need for this activity:

- Paper and pen or note-taking phone app

- Peaceful and comfortable space

- Fifteen to twenty minutes of dedicated time

INSTRUCTIONS

1. Stand, lie down, or sit comfortably in any position.

2. Set up any sounds or smells that bring comfort.

3. Read the list-making prompt, then write down at least three responses (they can be a few words or full sentences).

4. Alternatively, consider recording audio or video answers if note-taking is not your jam.

Make a list of:

- Things that make my body move differently

- Things that help me calm down

- Things that help me wake TF up

- Things I can do right now for better sleep

- Things I can try later for better sleep

- Things that stress me out every week

- Ways I can better nourish my body today

- Ways I can better nourish my body next week

Need a little help? Here's my list:

- Things that make my body move differently:

    - Brain fog makes me less sharp

    - Hypermobile spaghetti joints

    - Pesky muscle spasms

- Things that help me calm down:

    - Screaming, humming, or singing out loud

    - Taking a brisk walk

    - Squeezing all my muscles and then relaxing them

- Things that help me wake TF up:
    - Turning on the lights
    - Doing inversions and handstands
    - Fast, repetitive full-body exercises
- Things I can do right now for better sleep:
    - Go to sleep on time
    - Turn on night mode on devices
    - Do bed stretches and breathing exercises
- Things I can try later for better sleep:
    - Ask my partner about their snoring
    - Kick the dogs out of the bed
    - Buy a weighted blanket
- Things that stress me out every week:
    - Unexpected schedule changes and weather events
    - Health insurance denials and appeals
    - Meal preparation and planning
- Ways I can better nourish my body today:
    - Set reminders to eat
    - Pack extra water when I leave
    - Add a vegetable to dinner
- Ways I can better nourish my body next week:
    - Buy safe foods in bulk
    - Get frozen veggies
    - Set a reminder to buy the groceries

Movement Activity: Mobility Self-Assessment

We've assessed our sleep routines, nourishment habits, and mental road-blocks; now it's finally time to move our bodies. For this movement activity we'll take time to assess mobility at different joints. Joints require stability, which comes from muscle strength; and flexibility, which comes from muscle length. Testing different positions will tell a different story for either of those variables. For example, if you can't lift your arm toward the ceiling in an upright position (against gravity) but can achieve that motion while lying down, then it's a muscle-strength issue. You might choose to try each position for self-assessment or only the one that is accessible right now. You always have a choice. As all bodies are different, feel free to skip sections that don't apply to you. These movements may feel like a gentle warm-up for some or a full work-out for others. You're welcome to break this activity up over as many sessions, days, or weeks as you need. For example, you can take your time and focus on one section each week, or you can do multiple sections in one day. You can focus on only seated versions of assessments, or you can try them all but on different days. I'd recommend skimming ahead to see what's on paper and making a mental plan before getting physical.

For several joints, we will do full circles that combine movements to assess mobility. Keep in mind that they don't need to be perfect! I would also caution you not to force any of the movements. If you feel a hard stop, pause there and take notes. Also take notes on any differences between sides, funky motions, or achy spots. Don't worry too much about audible sounds, snaps, crackles, or pops unless pain accompanies those sounds. This assessment will help us in the next chapter as we start exploring movement and setting goals.

You can visit my website at www.MovementforEveryBody.org to find videos that accompany these instructions.

What you will need for this activity:

- Paper and pen or note-taking phone app

- Peaceful and comfortable space

- Fifteen to thirty minutes of dedicated time

- Optional mirror or phone to record for feedback

INSTRUCTIONS

1. Set up a comfy area to perform upright movements (whether sitting or standing), or lie down on the floor to do the movements.

2. If you're able to, set up a phone to record your movements, or position a mirror nearby.

3. Try two to three attempts of the movement as instructed.

4. Take notes on how each part of the movement made you feel.

ASSESSMENT INDEX

Assess the Neck

Chin Tucks Option A: Upright

1. Stand, kneel, or sit upright with a neutral spine.

2. Look straight ahead, with the chin parallel to the floor.

3. Without changing the position of the spine or shoulders, slide and tuck your chin back as far as you can.

4. Without changing the position of the spine or shoulders, slide and pull your chin forward as far as you can.

5. Return to the neutral starting position.

PRO TIPS

- Try visualizing a turkey gobble or a drawer sliding while performing the movement.

- You can also explore this movement while leaning against a wall with a soft ball or pillow behind your head.

- Take note if your head tilts or rotates unconsciously, or if there are any extra movements of the shoulder and upper back.

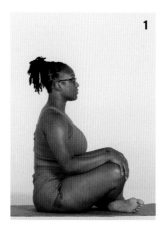 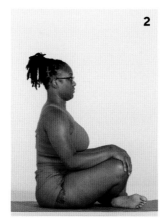 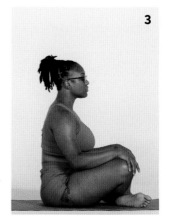

Chin Tucks Option B: Lying Down

1. Find a comfortable position on your belly, and lean on your elbows.

2. Look straight down, with the chin near perpendicular to the floor.

3. Without changing the position of the spine or shoulders, slide and tuck your chin up away from the floor.

4. Without changing the position of the spine or shoulders, slide and pull your chin down toward the floor.

5. Return to the neutral starting position.

PRO TIPS

- Try visualizing a turkey gobble or a drawer sliding while performing the movement.

- You can explore using blankets and pillows under the chest, belly, thighs, or ankles to add comfort.

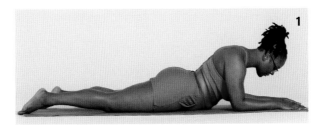

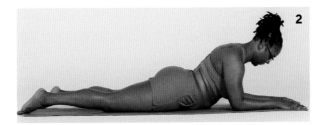

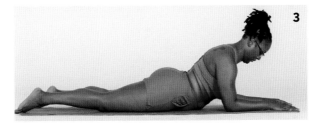

Neck Circles Option A: Upright

1. Stand, kneel, or sit upright with a neutral spine.

2. Bring your chin as close to your chest as possible, touching if you can.

3. Turn your head to the right, keeping the chin close to the chest.

4. Look up and to the right as you lift the head away from the right shoulder.

5. Look straight up as you rotate the head to the center.

6. Look up and to the left as you rotate and lower the head toward the left shoulder.

7. From here, look down as you turn the head back to center, keeping the chin close to the chest.

PRO TIPS

- To make the motion more fluid, imagine drawing a big circle with your chin.

- Take note if your head tilts or rotates unconsciously.

- Take note of any extra movements of the shoulder or upper back.

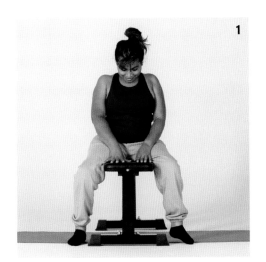

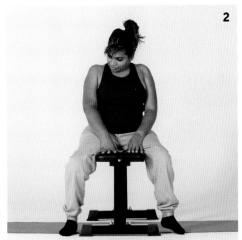

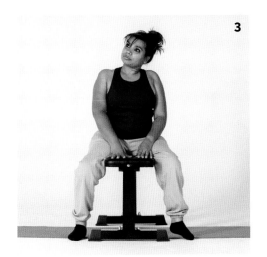

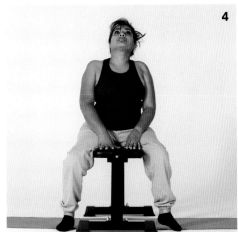

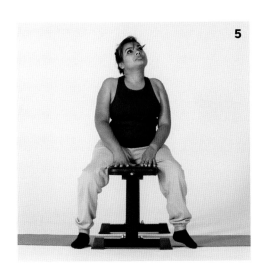

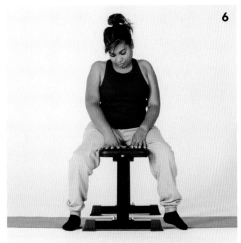

Neck Circles Option B: Lying Down

1. Find a comfortable position on your belly, and lean on your elbows.

2. Look straight down, with the chin near perpendicular to the floor.

3. Bring your chin as close to your chest as possible, touching if you can.

4. Turn your head to the left, keeping the chin close to the chest.

5. Look up and to the left as you lift the head away from the left shoulder.

6. Look straight up as you rotate the head to the center.

7. Look up and to the right as you rotate and lower the head toward the right shoulder.

8. From here, look down as you turn the head back to center, keeping the chin close to the chest.

PRO TIPS

- To make the motion more fluid, imagine drawing a big circle with your chin.

- You can explore using blankets and pillows under the chest, belly, thighs, or ankles to add comfort.

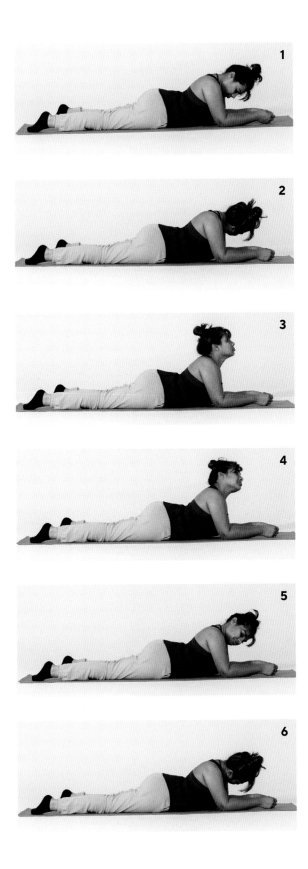

Assess the Spine

Spine Side Bends: Upright

1. Stand, kneel, or sit upright.

2. Make sure the spine and neck are neutral, and direct your gaze straight ahead.

3. Place your hands at your side, on your lap, on your hips, in the air, or behind your head.

4. Side bend to the right by bringing your right shoulder toward the floor.

5. Side bend to the left by bringing your left shoulder toward the floor.

PRO TIPS

▪ Feel free to explore all hand positions for this assessment.

▪ Take note of any extra spine rotation or bending in any direction.

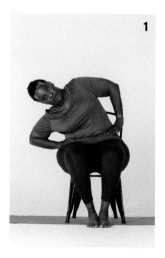 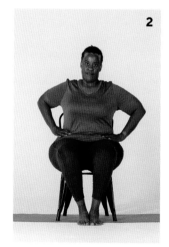 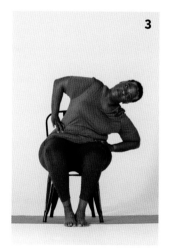

Spine Rotation Option A: Upright

1. Stand, kneel, or sit upright.

2. Make sure the spine and neck are neutral.

3. Place your hands at your side, on your lap, on your hips, in the air, or behind your head.

4. Rotate and twist to the right as far as is comfortable.

5. Return to center and take a few breaths.

6. Rotate and twist to the left as far as is comfortable.

PRO TIPS

- Note that breathing may feel more restricted while in a spinal twist.

- Avoid forcing more spine rotation by pulling with the arms.

- Be sure to keep the lower body planted for this motion.

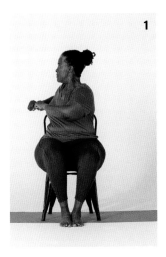 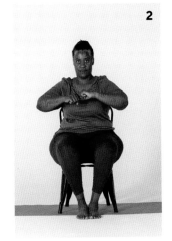 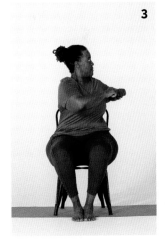

Spine Rotation Option B: Hands and Knees

1. Get on your hands and knees on the floor, a firm mattress, or a sturdy couch.

2. Make sure the knees are directly under the hip joints and spaced about hip distance apart.

3. Make sure the arms are directly under the shoulder joints and spaced shoulder distance apart.

4. Make sure the spine and neck are neutral, and direct your gaze downward between your arms.

5. Lift the right arm to the ceiling as you rotate the spine to the right as far as is comfortable.

   - Or place the right hand behind your head and lift the right elbow to the ceiling.

6. Lift the left arm to the ceiling as you rotate the spine to the left as far as is comfortable.

   - Or place the left hand behind your head and lift the left elbow to the ceiling.

PRO TIPS

- Take note of any extra movements of the hips or of the arm that's in contact with the surface.

- For most movements in the hands-and-knees position, you can also rest the supporting arm on a chair, stool, or stack of yoga blocks versus placing the hand flat on the floor.

- Feel free to explore both hand positions for this assessment or to skip lifting the arms entirely.

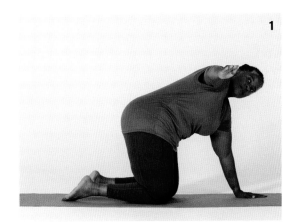

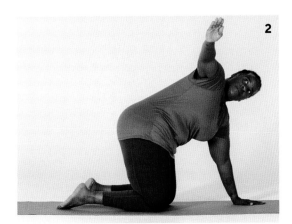

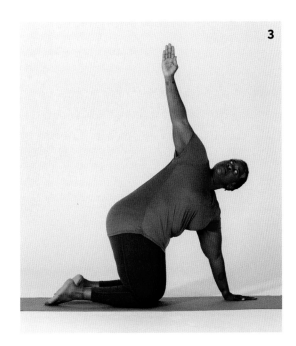

Cat and Cow (Marjaryasana/Bitilasana) Option A: Upright

1. Stand, kneel, or sit upright.

2. Make sure the spine and neck are neutral, and direct your gaze straight ahead.

3. Place your hands at your side, on your lap, across your chest, or behind your head.

4. Try to perform the following movements without changing the position of the arms or the lower body:

   ■ Inhale and arch the entire spine as you look up toward the ceiling and lift the chin away from your chest.

   ■ Exhale and curl the entire spine as you look toward your belly button and pull the chin toward your chest.

PRO TIPS

■ Feel free to explore all hand positions for this assessment.

■ If this motion goes smoothly, try a segmental version by moving one spine bone at a time instead of everything all at once.

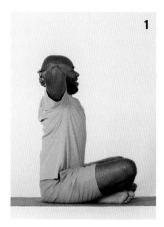
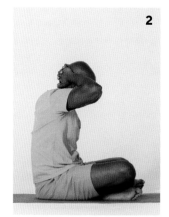
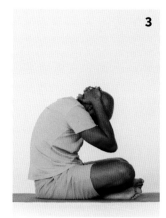

Cat and Cow (Marjaryasana/Bitilasana) Option B: Hands and Knees

1. Get on your hands and knees on the floor, a firm mattress, or a sturdy couch.

2. Make sure the knees are directly under the hip joints and spaced about hip distance apart.

3. Make sure the arms are directly under the shoulder joints and spaced shoulder distance apart.

4. Make sure the spine and neck are neutral, and direct your gaze down between your arms.

5. Try to perform the following movements without changing the position of the head or elbows:

   ▪ Inhale and arch the entire spine as you look up toward the ceiling and pull the chin away from your chest.

   ▪ Exhale and curl the entire spine as you look toward your belly button and pull the chin toward your chest.

6. Relax back to neutral position.

PRO TIPS

▪ If you have trouble keeping the arms straight as you move, go for the bent-elbow option. Rest the elbows on stacked yoga blocks or books.

▪ If this motion goes smoothly, try a segmental version by moving one spine bone at a time instead of everything all at once.

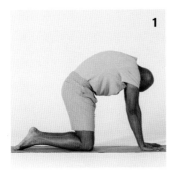 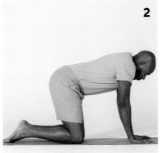 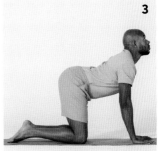

Pelvic Tilts Option A: Upright

1. Stand, kneel, or sit upright.

2. Make sure the spine and neck are neutral, and direct your gaze straight ahead.

3. Try to perform the following movements without changing the position of the upper back:

   ▪ Arch the lower back and push the belly out to anterior pelvic tilt.

   ▪ Curl the lower back and pull the belly in to posterior pelvic tilt.

PRO TIPS

▪ You can place your hands on your sides—above the hip, right on the pelvis bone—for more feedback on position.

▪ If balance isn't a concern, sitting on a ball can help make this motion more fluid.

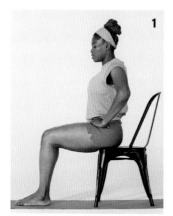 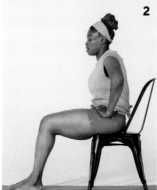 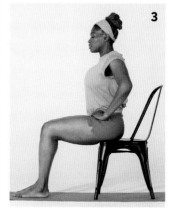

Pelvic Tilts Option B: Hands and Knees

1. Get on your hands and knees on the floor, a firm mattress, or a couch.

2. Make sure the knees are directly under the hip joints and spaced about hip distance apart.

3. Make sure the arms are directly under the shoulder joints and spaced shoulder distance apart.

4. Make sure the spine and neck are neutral, and direct your gaze down between your arms.

5. Try to perform the following movements without changing the position of the arms or upper back:

   ▪ Sink the lower back down toward the floor to anterior pelvic tilt.

   ▪ Lift the lower back up toward the ceiling to posterior pelvic tilt.

PRO TIPS

▪ These movements look simple, but it can be tough to isolate them.

▪ Some folks rest naturally in anterior or posterior pelvic tilt. Muscle tightness can also affect resting pelvis positioning.

▪ If getting on your hands and knees is uncomfortable, you can also assess this motion while lying on your back.

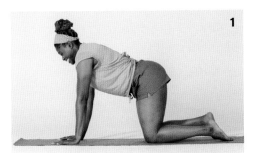

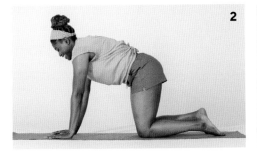
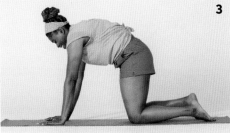

Assess the Shoulders

Scapular Circles Option A: Upright

1. Stand, kneel, or sit upright.

2. Make sure the spine and neck are neutral, and direct your gaze straight ahead.

3. Raise one or both arms to shoulder level.

4. Try to perform the following movements without changing the position of the neck, elbows, and spine:

   ▪ First, pull your arms forward for scapular protraction.

   ▪ Second, pull your shoulder blades up toward your ears for scapular elevation.

   ▪ Next, squeeze your shoulder blades back and together for scapular retraction.

   ▪ Then, pull your shoulder blades back and down for scapular depression.

PRO TIPS

▪ You can try straight arms with hands free or holding a light object like a book or yoga block.

▪ If you have trouble keeping the arms straight as you move, bend the elbows at a ninety-degree angle.

1

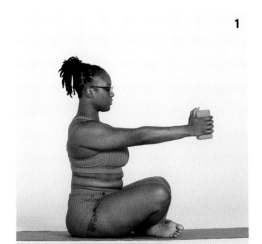

2

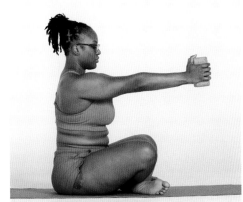

3

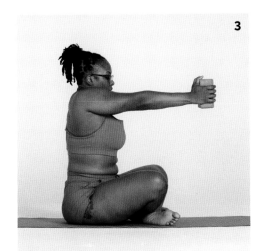

4

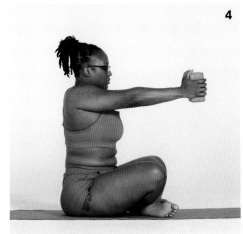

5

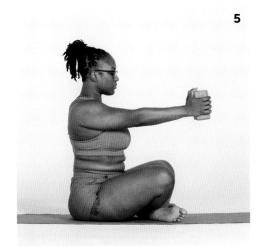

6

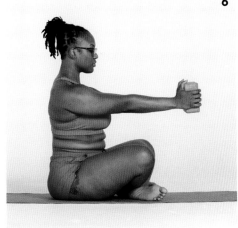

Scapular Circles Option B: Hands and Knees

1. Get on your hands and knees on the floor, a firm mattress, or a sturdy couch.

2. Make sure the knees are directly under the hip joints and spaced about hip distance apart.

3. Make sure the arms are directly under the shoulder joints and spaced shoulder distance apart.

4. Make sure the spine and neck are neutral, and direct your gaze down between your arms.

5. Try to perform the following movements without changing the position of the elbows, hands, lower spine, or legs:

   - First, push away from the floor for scapular protraction.

   - Second, pull your shoulder blades down toward your bottom for scapular depression.

   - Next, sink down toward the floor for scapular retraction.

   - Then, pull your shoulder blades up toward your ears for scapular elevation.

PRO TIPS

- You can try straight arms with hands on the level surface or resting on your fists.

- If you have trouble keeping the arms straight as you move, go for the bent-elbow option. Rest the elbows on stacked yoga blocks or books.

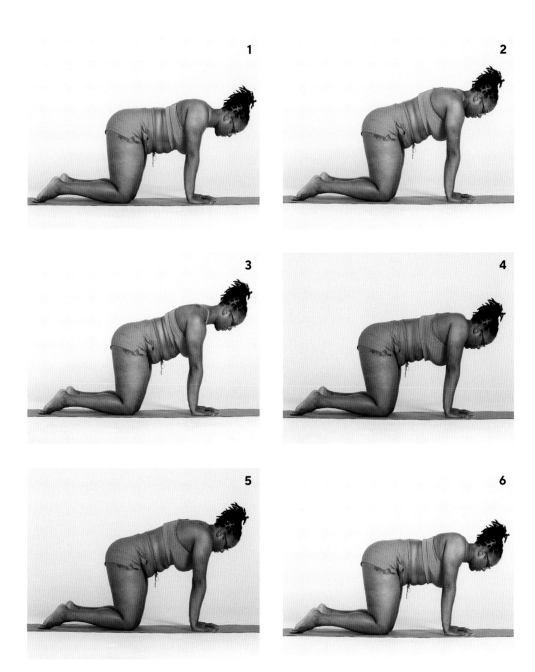

Shoulder Circles Option A: Upright

1. Stand, kneel, or sit upright in an armless chair.

2. First, drop one arm straight down your side, with the palm facing your body.

3. Second, lift that arm until it's over your head, with the elbow near your ear. Your thumb will go from pointing up to pointing backward, with the palm turned toward your face.

4. Next, rotate the arm so that the palm turns away from your face.

5. Then, as you lower the arm behind you, continue to rotate the arm until the palm is turned toward your face and the thumb points forward.

6. Finally, lower the arm down at your side to reset.

PRO TIPS

- Pay attention to any compensatory (i.e., extra) rotation of the spine.

- You can explore this upright version while leaning against a wall to limit spine movement.

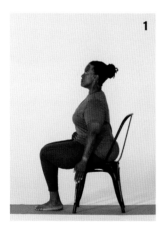
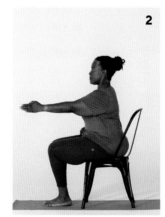
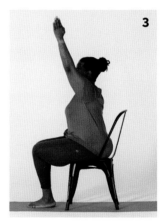
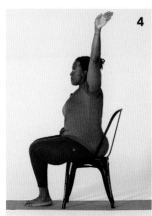
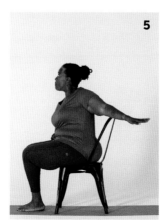
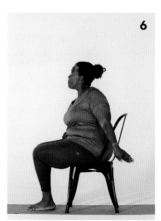

Shoulder Circles Option B: Lying Down

1. Lie down on your side in a comfortable position.

2. First, reach forward with the top arm, keeping the arm parallel to the floor and the palm facing down.

3. Second, move the top arm over your head so that the elbow is near your ear.

4. Next, rotate the top arm so that the palm faces up.

5. Then, as you move the top arm directly behind you, continue to rotate the arm until the palm faces down again.

6. Finally, pull the top arm over your side and back to the starting position.

PRO TIPS

- Pay attention to any compensatory (i.e., extra) rotation of the spine or hips.

- Use cushions and blankets for comfort at the head or shoulder, or between the legs, if needed.

- You may choose to lean on an elbow to lie down completely on your side.

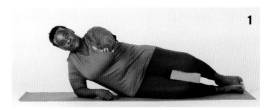

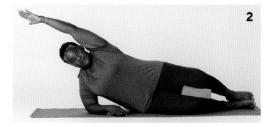

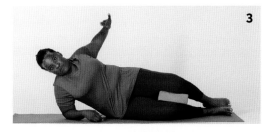

Shoulder Movement Screen Option A: Upright

1. Stand, kneel, or sit upright.

2. Move one arm at a time, or try both as shown.

3. Take one hand, and with the palm facing forward, reach behind your head. If you reach, try to walk the fingers down a little lower on the spine. If doing both arms at the same time, see if you can touch the other hand.

   ▪ This combines flexion, abduction, horizontal abduction, and external rotation.

4. Take one hand (or the second hand for two at a time), and with the palm facing backward, reach for your lower back. If you reach, try to inch the fingers up toward the head. If doing both arms at the same time, see if you can touch the other hand.

   ▪ This combines extension, adduction, horizontal abduction, and internal rotation.

PRO TIPS

   ▪ Pay attention to any compensatory (i.e., extra) neck or back movements.

   ▪ If there are several compensatory movements, do one arm at a time.

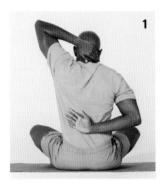
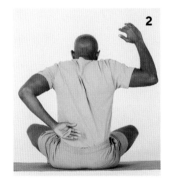
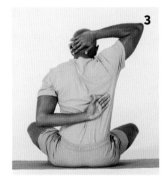
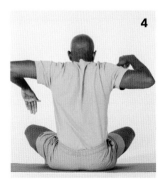
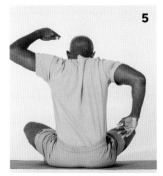
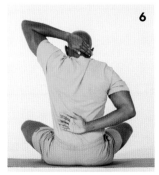

Shoulder Movement Screen Option B: Lying Down

1. Lie down on your side in a comfortable position.

2. Take one hand, and with the palm facing backward, reach for your lower back. If you reach, try to inch the fingers up toward the head.

   - This combines extension, adduction, horizontal abduction, and internal rotation.

3. Take one hand, and with the palm facing forward, reach behind your head. If you reach, try to walk the fingers down a little lower on the spine.

   - This combines flexion, abduction, horizontal abduction, and external rotation.

PRO TIPS

- Pay attention to any compensatory (i.e., extra) neck or back movements.

- Use cushions and blankets for comfort at the head or shoulder, or between the legs, if needed.

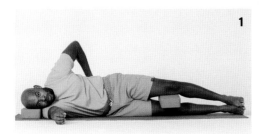
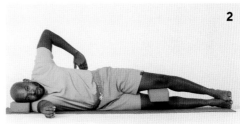
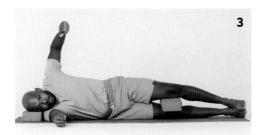
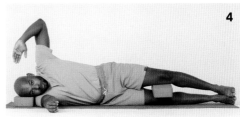
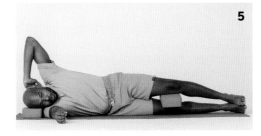
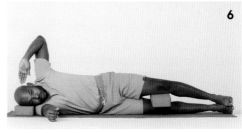

Assess the Elbows, Wrists, and Hands

Elbow Flexion and Extension: Upright

1. Stand, kneel, or sit upright.

2. Drop your arms at your side, with the palms facing forward.

3. Bend your elbows, aiming to bring your palms as close to the shoulder as possible.

4. Lower the arms and return to start, straightening as much as possible.

PRO TIPS

■ This movement can also be assessed while lying down.

■ If your arm seems to straighten *too* much (mine do!), that's called elbow hyperextension.

■ If you have trouble turning the palms up, we will explore that specific movement next.

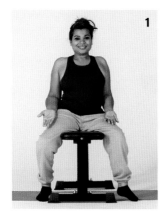 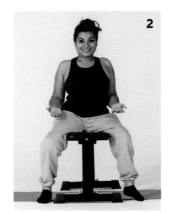 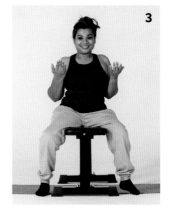

Elbow Supination and Pronation (Rotation): Upright

1. Stand, kneel, or sit upright.

   ■ If standing, bend your arms at the elbow until the forearms are parallel with the floor.

   ■ If seated, rest the backs of your hands on your lap, a pillow, a book, or a yoga block.

2. Rotate the hands so that the palms are facing down, without changing the elbow position.

3. Rotate the hands so that the palms are facing up, without changing the elbow position.

PRO TIPS

■ Rotation happens at the elbow and the wrist joint. Limitations can come from either area.

■ Pay attention to extra elbow movements. Try not to flex or extend the elbow while rotating.

■ This movement can also be assessed while lying on your back with your elbows bent at a ninety-degree angle.

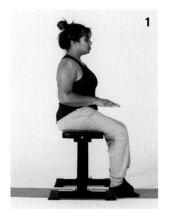 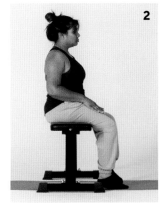 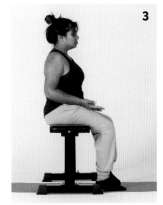

Wrist Circles Palm Up: Upright

1. Stand, kneel, or sit upright.

   ◾ If standing, bend at the elbows until the forearms are parallel with the floor.

   ◾ If seated, rest the backs of your forearms on your lap, a pillow, a book, or a yoga block.

2. First, make fists and turn your palms up toward the ceiling.

3. Second, pull your knuckles up toward your face to flex the wrists against gravity.

4. Next, pull the knuckles outward to radially deviate the wrists as you lower the fists to the starting position.

5. Then, pull the knuckles toward the floor to extend the wrists.

6. From here, pull the knuckles inward to ulnarly deviate the wrists as you bring the fists back up to the starting position.

PRO TIPS

◾ This rotation for this movement happens only at the wrist joint.

◾ Pay attention to extra movements, and try not to rotate at the elbow joint.

◾ Explore squeezing a towel at your side for the standing version.

◾ This movement can also be assessed while lying on your back with your elbows bent at a ninety-degree angle.

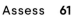

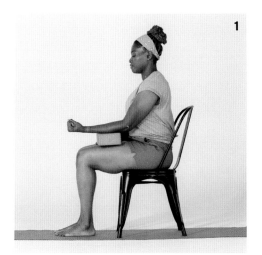

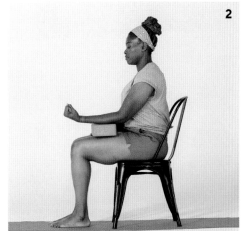

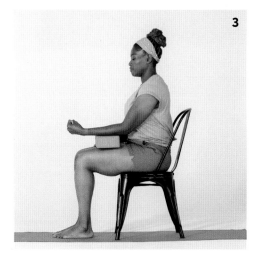

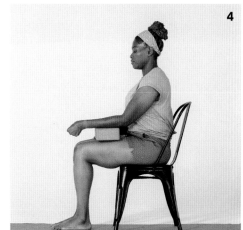

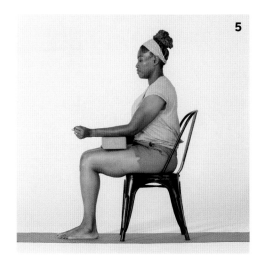

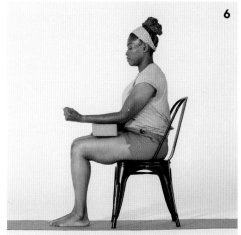

Wrist Circles Palm Down: Upright

1. Stand, kneel, or sit upright.

   ■ If standing, bend at the elbows until the forearms are parallel with the floor.

   ■ If seated, rest the backs of your forearms on your lap, a pillow, a book, or a yoga block.

2. First, make fists and turn your palms down toward the floor.

3. Second, pull your knuckles up toward your face to extend the wrists against gravity.

4. Next, pull the knuckles outward to ulnarly deviate the wrists as you lower the fists to the starting position.

5. Then, pull the knuckles toward the floor to flex the wrists.

6. From here, pull the knuckles inward to radially deviate the wrists as you bring the fists back up to the starting position.

PRO TIPS

■ The rotation for this movement happens only at the wrist joint.

■ Pay attention to extra movements, and try not to rotate at the elbow joint.

■ Explore squeezing a towel at your side for the standing version.

■ This movement can also be assessed while lying on your back with elbows bent at a ninety-degree angle.

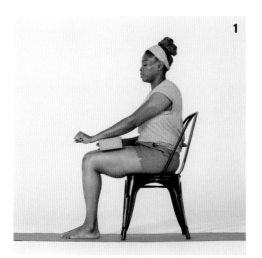

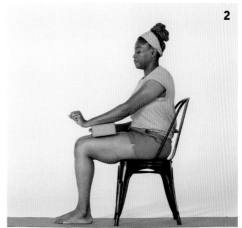

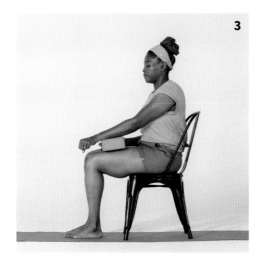

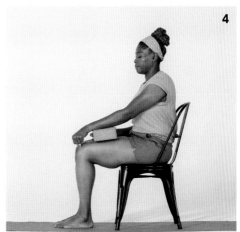

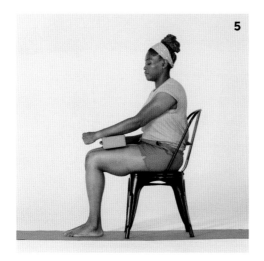

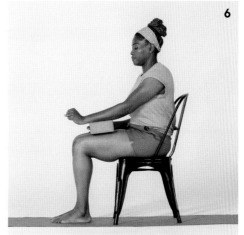

Finger Abduction/Adduction (Open/Close): Any Position

1. Assume a comfortable starting position lying down, sitting, or standing.

   ▪ If standing, bend the arms at the elbow until the forearms are parallel with the floor.

   ▪ If seated, rest the backs of your forearms on your lap, a pillow, a book, or a yoga block.

   ▪ If lying down, keep the elbows bent at a ninety-degree angle.

2. First, with an open hand and straight fingers, turn your palms upward.

3. Second, squeeze the fingers together for three to five seconds.

4. Next, squeeze the fingers apart for three to five seconds.

5. Repeat a few cycles, and take note of any cramps or fatigue.

PRO TIPS

▪ Feel free to focus on one side at a time if the movement is difficult.

▪ It's common to have difference between the dominant side and the nondominant side.

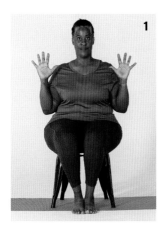
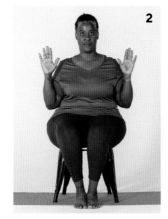
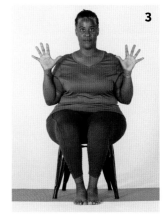

Finger Opposition: Any Position

1. Assume a comfortable starting position lying down, sitting, or standing.

   - If standing, bend the arms at the elbow until the forearms are parallel with the floor.

   - If seated, rest the backs of your forearms on your lap, a pillow, a book, or a yoga block.

   - If lying down, keep the elbow bent at a ninety-degree angle.

2. Start with an open hand and straight fingers, and turn your palm upward.

3. Touch the tip of the thumb to the tip of the index finger, then rest.

4. Touch the tip of the thumb to the tip of the middle finger, then rest.

5. Touch the tip of the thumb to the tip of the ring finger, then rest.

6. Touch the tip of the thumb to the tip of the pinky finger, then rest.

7. Repeat a few cycles, and take note of any cramps or fatigue.

PRO TIPS

- Feel free to touch fingertips at the top edges to form a circle (harder) or at the finger pads with the fingers straight (easier).

- You can also use your other hand to help the fingers complete the movement if they don't reach; then see if you can hold the squeeze.

- It's common to have difference between the dominant side and the nondominant side.

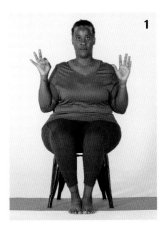 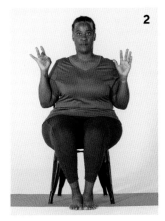 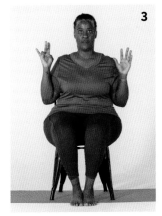

Assess the Hips and Knees

Hip Circles Option A: Standing Upright

1. Stand tall, with the legs about hip distance apart and a neutral spine.

2. Lift one leg up as high as you can with a bent knee.

3. Rotate the hip outward so that the lower leg moves toward the standing leg.

4. From this height and position, swing the whole leg out to the side as far as you can.

5. Rotate the hip inward so that the lower leg moves backward, then kick back as far as comfortable with a bent knee.

6. Lower the whole leg toward the standing leg, with a bent knee.

7. Rest, and repeat on the other side if applicable.

PRO TIPS

■ Feel free to place one or two arms on a chair, wall, or table for extra support.

■ If lifting the leg is tough, break up the hip circles and take breaks in between.

■ For better balance practice your *drishti* (fixed gaze) by concentrating your gaze on a fixed spot in front of you.

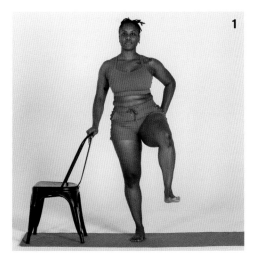

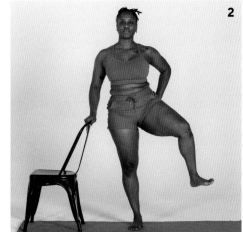

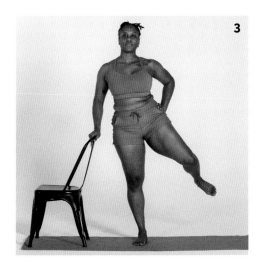

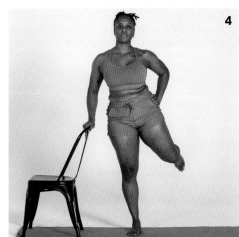

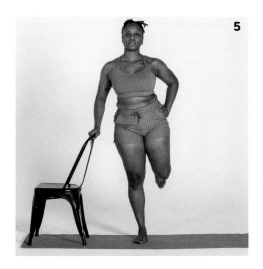

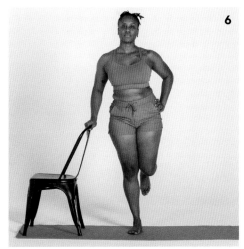

Hip Circles Option B: Seated Upright

1. Sit upright in an armless chair with a neutral spine.

2. Lift one leg with a bent knee as high as you can.

3. From this height and position, swing the whole leg out to the side as far as you can.

4. Rotate the hip inward so that the lower leg moves up toward the ceiling.

5. Bring the whole leg inward as you lower the knee down toward the floor and kick the whole leg backwards.

6. Lift the leg out to the side as high as you can.

7. Rotate the hip outward so that the lower leg moves toward you.

8. Swing the whole leg until it's in front of you.

9. Lower the leg and resume a resting position.

10. Rest and repeat on the other side if applicable.

PRO TIPS

■ Feel free to place one or two arms on another chair, wall, or table for extra support.

■ You can also explore holding the arms forward with fisted hands or holding onto a block.

■ If lifting the leg is tough, take a break with the knee lowered to the floor before completing the circle.

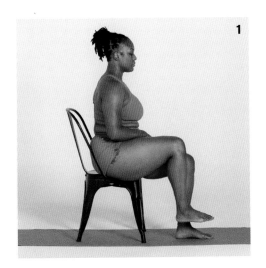

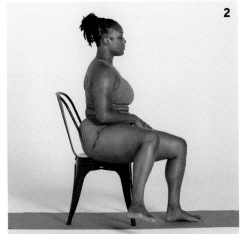

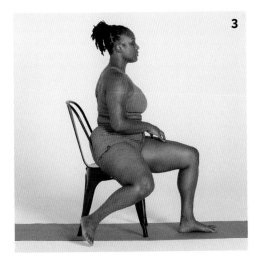

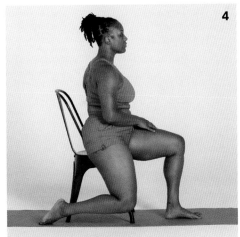

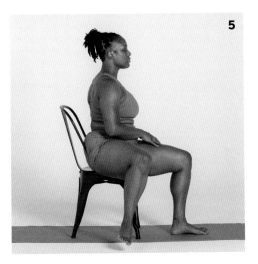

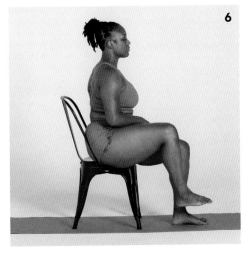

Knee Flexion and Extension Option A: Upright

1. Sit upright in a chair with the legs about hip distance apart and feet on the ground.

2. Slide one foot backward and bend that knee as much as you can.

3. Reset to starting position.

4. Lift the same leg upward from the knee, straightening that knee as much as you can.

5. Reset to starting position. Rest and repeat on the other side if applicable.

PRO TIPS

▪ If it brings comfort, go ahead and lean back into that chair.

▪ If you need more room to slide and lift, try yoga blocks or a book underneath the thigh.

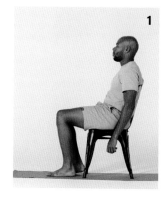 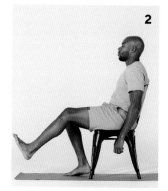 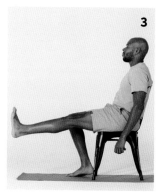

Knee Flexion and Extension Option B: Lying Down

1. Lie down on your back, with a neutral spine and knees bent.

2. Use your hands, a strap, a belt, or a rolled sheet to support the back of one leg as you lift the knee toward your chest until the thigh is perpendicular to the floor.

3. From this position, straighten the knee as much as you can.

PRO TIPS

- If you can't straighten the knee in this position, that can be from hamstring muscle tightness.

- If you can straighten the knee without a problem, you can explore straightening the opposite knee.

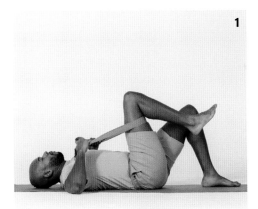

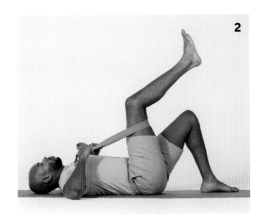

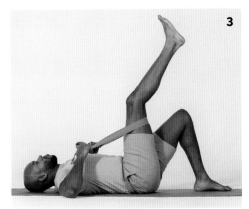

Knee Rotation with Foot Down: Upright

1. Sit upright in a chair, with the legs about hip distance apart and feet on the ground.

2. Bend one knee to about ninety degrees, with the foot facing forward.

3. Try to perform the following movements without changing the position of the hips, knee, or heel:

   - With the heel planted, rotate the knee inward by lifting the toes and bringing them toward the other leg.

   - With the heel planted, rotate the knee outward by lifting the toes and turning them away from the other leg.

PRO TIPS

- If it brings comfort, go ahead and lean back into that chair.

- The knee does not rotate as much as the hips, shoulders, and wrists.

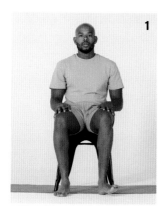 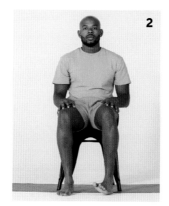 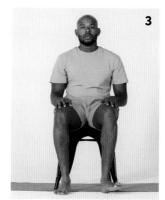

Knee Rotation with Foot Up: Upright

1. Sit upright in a chair with the legs about hip distance apart and feet on the ground.

2. Bend one knee to about ninety degrees with the foot facing forward.

3. Lift this leg and hold at this height. Try to perform the following movements without changing the position of the hips or knee:

   - With the foot up, rotate the knee inward by bringing the toes toward the other leg.

   - With the foot up, rotate the knee outward by turning the toes away from the other leg.

PRO TIPS

- If it brings comfort, go ahead and lean back into that chair.

- It may be harder to isolate knee rotation from foot and ankle motion with this option.

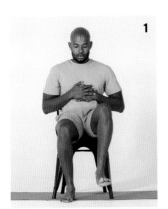 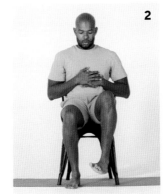 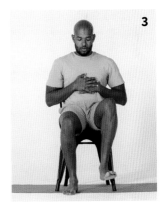

Assess the Ankles and Feet

Ankle Circles Option A: Upright

1. Assume a comfortable upright starting position, sitting or standing.

2. From either position, lift one leg to a comfortable height you can maintain.

3. Try to perform the following movements without changing the position of the hip or knee:

   ■ First, start with the foot parallel to the floor.

   ■ Second, turn the foot and toes inward.

   ■ Next, lift the foot and toes up as high as you can toward your face.

   ■ Then, turn the foot and toes outward.

   ■ Finally, point the foot and toes as far down as you can.

PRO TIPS

■ To make this motion more fluid, imagine drawing a circle with your big toe.

■ If lifting and holding the height are difficult, try the seated option with a yoga block or a book under the thigh.

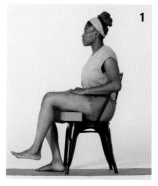
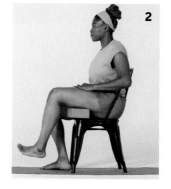
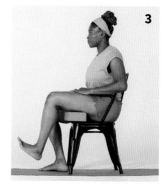
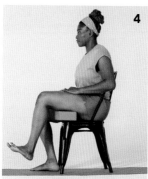
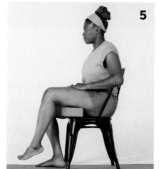
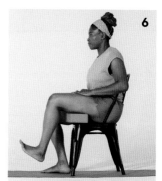

Ankle Circles Option B: Lying Down

1. Lie down on your back with a neutral spine and knees bent or straight.

2. Use your hands, a strap, a belt, or a rolled sheet to support the back of one leg as you lift the knee toward your chest until the thigh is perpendicular to the floor.

3. Try to perform the following movements without changing the position of the hip or knee:

   - First, start with the foot parallel to the floor.

   - Second, turn the foot and toes inward.

   - Next, lift the foot and toes up as high as you can toward your face.

   - Then, turn the foot and toes outward.

   - Finally, point the foot and toes as far down as you can.

PRO TIPS

- To make this motion more fluid, imagine drawing a circle on the ceiling with your big toe.

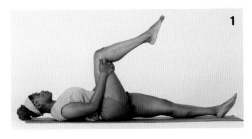 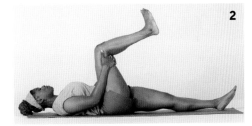

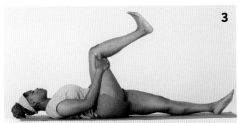 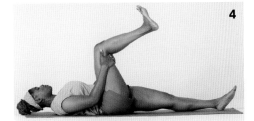

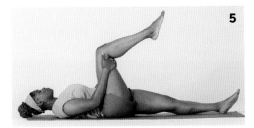 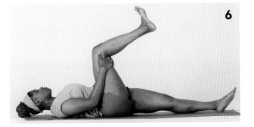

Toe Flexion and Extension: Any Position

1. Assume a comfortable starting position lying down, sitting, or standing.

   ▪ If standing or sitting, lift one leg to a comfortable height.

   ▪ If lying down, lift the knee toward the chest and support the thigh with hands, a yoga block, or a strap.

2. Try to perform the following movements without changing the position of the hip, knee, or ankle:

   ▪ Pull your toes up toward your nose.

   ▪ Curl your toes down away from your nose.

PRO TIPS

▪ If lifting the leg and holding at a comfortable height are difficult, try the seated option with a yoga block or book under the thigh.

▪ If lifting and holding are okay but balance is hard, feel free to place one or two arms on a chair, wall, or table for extra support.

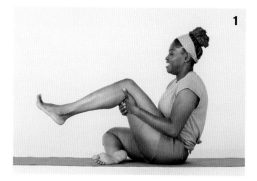

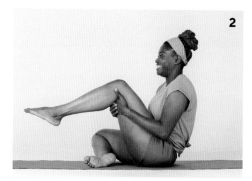

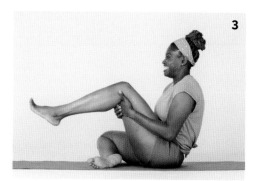

Explore

What Do We Need to Explore?

As we reach the exploration phase of this adventure, it's time to start expanding and stretching ourselves. If this book is a road map, we've finished deliberating where we want to go and choosing a destination. We discovered a few routes to get there, and now it's time to start moving toward our destination of achieving something tangible. We've appraised and unpacked toxic fitness nonsense, then assessed and reviewed our current abilities and thoughts. We are now ready to figure out how we need to move in order to reach our goals. This is the part of the journey where questions are asked, and only you can know the answer. This part of the journey will still require some measure of journaling, logging, tracking, and retrospection as we lead ourselves forward with compassion and curiosity.

Exploring How We Move

As we explore, we must understand how to view exercise and practice discernment to choose what might work. We must be able to discern what isn't right for us without feeling ashamed or engaging in negative self-talk. Unless you're working closely with a knowledgeable personal trainer, a licensed physical therapist, or some other trained movement professional, you're likely turning to the internet for advice. The internet is chock-full of information that can be hard to sort through. But I promise you this: remembering that *nobody* knows your body better than you will make it easier to sort through the noise. No influencer, no cool guy on YouTube, nobody with hundreds of thousands of followers can teach you how to move your body the best. Everything you find online is a recommendation, a suggestion, an option. It's up to you to decide how to fit that option into your life.

Put yourself first and keep yourself in mind as you explore workouts and dive into the deep oceans of information on the internet. Instead of comparison or shame, start with curiosity. Ask yourself questions to determine whether general advice may be personalized to your individual needs. Here are a few questions that may help you practice that discernment:

- What kind of person is this account making exercises for?

- Does this person seem to offer lots of options for different shapes and abilities?

- What is the purpose of this exercise?

- How could I break down this whole exercise into smaller parts?

- How could I take the main idea of this exercise but change the setup?

- Where would I need more support?

- Where would I need less support?

- Is this intense for me, or is it pretty chill?

- If it's too intense, how can I turn down the knob?

- If it's too chill, how can I turn up the heat?

Exploring When We Move

We might be able to figure out how to make movements work, how to choose props and options that are appropriate for our needs, and whom to follow on the internet for useful advice. But what about the timing? When do we move? How much do we move? How can we avoid the sense of doing too little? How do we break the all-or-nothing cycle of doing too much or absolutely nothing? How can we avoid becoming bored or burdened by exercise? The answer depends, of course, but there are plenty of options to explore what would work best.

First we have to figure out which method of planning works best for our physical demands, mental bandwidth, available time, and access. For some people, planning out their workouts at the beginning of the week works well. For others, making a monthly schedule makes more sense. Hiring a movement professional or physical therapist to assist with exercise planning can be helpful if you have access to one.

Next, explore whether you enjoy movement early in the morning, on a full or empty stomach, late at night, or even during lunch breaks. Consider how much time you need to transition between activities, spaces, and tasks. Determine whether you are a "I do all my tasks outside and only relax when I get home" person, a "I'd rather exercise at home on my own" person, or even an "I hate working out alone" person. Maybe you're all of them, depending on the activity. Dive into that!

Finally, determine which tools are useful for memory cues and time management. This can make a huge difference. Perhaps you add movement to your physical or phone calendar. You might find it useful to plan out your week on a large dry-erase board. Sometimes keeping track of tutorials is easier with a social media account dedicated to only bookmarking exercises. You might find it useful to have an accountability partner or to use an app to record your activity.

Here's a list of external memory cues, practices, and ideas to get you started:

- Timers, calendars, stickers/sticky notes, dry-erase boards, printed routines/checklists

- Accountability buddy, online groups, fitness app communities

- Fitness app, diary and journal apps, physical diary, physical exercise journal

It's also important to understand how to free ourselves from an all-or-nothing binary. Consistent effort yields consistent results. But what exactly does consistency mean? Is this a term that requires exploration, deconstruction, and reclamation? Contrary to what a toxic fitness influencer may say, consistency does not mean "no pain, no gain." Consistency is not equivalent to pushing yourself to your limits every time you work out—you have other options than "burn yourself out just to say you exercised" and "rest for months before returning to exercise." There's a lot in between! Consistency is really about understanding that doing a small amount for a long time can make a big difference. Consistency is all about being constant in showing up for yourself with nourishment, grace, and compassion. This showing up involves understanding what you can handle on your best and worst days. It means recognizing that something can be better than nothing. It's useful to know what bare minimums you can achieve on a low-battery day because if you choose movement that drains you or choose nothing at all and never find yourself moving again, you lose either way. There can be no growth if we are stuck in a cycle of shooting for the moon when we feel well, then crashing and burning whenever we don't. You may also need to rethink what the "something" is that's better than nothing in these situations. Is it swapping a gym lift with a longer dog walk? Practicing breathwork on the couch at home instead of driving to the Pilates studio? All of these swaps of something for nothing foster consistency.

Example: When We Move

Let's tie it all together with an example. Of course, keep in mind that nobody can totally figure any of this out for you but you.

Let's say you'd like to work on mobility, yoga, and barbell movements while working and caregiving full time. At the start of each week, you open your phone calendar to see what's going on for the next seven days. You think about work tasks, caregiving demands, and general adulting required for the week. On a dry-erase board you write down the happenings for each day, and you decide which days are best for grocery shopping, cooking, and going to the gym for barbell exercises. You pick "easier" days when you have support available or the time to drive somewhere extra. You build yoga flows into your daily routine with a family-friendly ten-minute routine everyone can do together before dinner. You build mobility into your sleep hygiene/bedtime routine by adding five minutes of chill mobility exercises to do before bed. Your bedtime routine is a printed checklist on your bathroom mirror so you don't forget any of the steps. On the bare-minimum days, you could skip yoga in favor of a longer chill mobility session before bed. On days when you have an unexpected shift or demand, such as a sick child or a flat tire, you might skip the gym and do bodyweight exercises at home. Of course, napping or completely resting is always an option.

Exploring when and how to move is also easier with goals in mind!

Exploring Why We Move

Having a specific goal in mind often helps give meaning to either joyful move-ment or routines that boost joyful movement. What's the difference? Well, all movement does not have to be joyful, but all movement should be intentional. Joyful movement usually entails an embodiment practice chosen based on activities and environments that spark joy, curiosity, and exploration. The movement is chosen because it offers joy, regardless of the environment or demands. Will this hold true for all physical activities? Of course not!

You may enjoy running indoors on the treadmill or hiking with friends out-doors for different reasons. But with either example, a focus on boring core sta-bilization, hip mobility, and ankle-strength exercises could improve the quality of those movements or mitigate injuries. You might choose to do Pilates via in-person group classes and do kettlebell workouts alone at home. With either example, you might need to work separately on tedious wrist-strengthening exercises to support either activity. Every movement you make may not be enjoyable, but every movement you make should be intentional, in the sense that you should know why you're doing it and what you want to achieve.

For example, I enjoy barbell sports and am currently in love with Olym-pic weightlifting, which necessitates a high level of overhead stability, control, technique, and awareness. As a hypermobile klutz with weak proprioception (awareness of my body parts in space), I lack all of these abilities. I enjoy weight-lifting, and I understand that to continue enjoying it, I will have to engage in movements I don't enjoy such as rotator cuff strengthening and boring core stabilization work. The intention is clear: I want to lower my chances of injuring myself while doing something I like.

Setting Smart Goals

Now that we understand how to choose and plan movement, we need to set the intention for movement by making goals. They don't have to be huge, but they do have to be SMART:

S	M	A	R	T
Specific	Measurable	Attainable	Relevant	Time based

To create a *specific* goal, ask:

- What movement do you want to achieve?

- What are all the variables you'll need to consider?

To create a *measurable* goal, ask:

- How will you know the goal was achieved?

- What quantifiable outcome or objective measure can be used?

To create an *attainable* goal, ask:

- What movement is realistic and achievable?

- Which movement do you have the foundational skills for?

To create a *relevant* goal, ask:

- Why does it matter if this movement is achieved?

- Which is the focus, improving function or bringing joy?

To create a *time-based* goal, ask:

- When can you achieve this?

- How will you define the target time frame or deadline?

With a SMART goal in mind, choosing movement and making a plan might make a little more sense. Here are more questions to keep in mind with your SMART goal setting and even smarter exercise planning:

- What do I need to work on to achieve this goal?

- How can I break up this goal into small chunks?

- How much time can I commit to these movements in the long run?

- What does the final outcome look like? How is it measured?

- What happens if I don't meet this outcome?

- Should I take pictures or video?

- How will I record my work and progress?

Here are a few examples of a SMART goal and SMART plan in action:

Goal: I want to stand up from the floor without struggling.

SMART goal: In four months, I'll stand up from the floor without using my hands on the first try.

SMART plan: I will work on lower body strengthening and core work for at least ten minutes at a time, twice a week. At least once a month I will practice getting up from the floor.

Goal: I hate that I'm out of breath when I walk my dog.

SMART goal: In two months, I'll walk ten minutes at a fast pace without getting winded.

SMART plan: I'll end every walk by walking at a brisk pace for at least two minutes, adding time as it gets easier.

Goal: I wish my elbow didn't hurt during rock climbing.

SMART goal: In six weeks, my elbow pain while rock climbing will go from a 6 on a 10-point scale to a 3 on a 10-point scale.

SMART plan: I will work on hand and wrist strength exercises twice a week for ten minutes at a time, and I'll do daily wrist and shoulder stretches for five minutes per day.

Journaling Activity: Make SMART Goals

Whether we want to improve the quality of joyful movement or of everyday functioning, we must always "begin with the end in mind," as Stephen Covey says in *The 7 Habits of Highly Effective People*. Having a specific, measurable, attainable, relevant, and time-based goal will help to guide this journey and exploration of movement. As you prepare to create these goals, keep in mind that the process can be as tactile or visual as you desire, as practical or whimsical as you like. You can write goals in a paper notebook with different-colored pens and highlighters and use a calendar with stickers to keep track. Alternatively, you might scribble down some notes in your notes app and capture videos in a stored album on your phone. Consider what level of effort and access works best for your brain.

What you will need for this activity:

■ Paper and pen or note-taking phone app

■ Peaceful and comfortable space

■ Fifteen to twenty minutes of dedicated time

INSTRUCTIONS

1. Stand, lie down, or sit comfortably in any position.

2. Set up any sounds or smells that bring comfort.

3. In the steps below, read each prompt, then note your responses.

4. Alternatively, consider recording audio or video answers if note-taking is not your jam.

Step 1: Make a List

■ Specific exercises that you enjoy

■ Specific exercises that you struggle with

■ Areas of pain and stiffness in your body

■ Areas of discomfort and instability in your body

■ Your current season of joyful movement practices

■ Mobility and function needed for above joyful movement practices

Step 2: Review the List

■ Which points stick out to you the most?

■ Which areas are most important in your life right now?

■ Which of these do you have time, energy, and access to work on?

Step 3: Craft your SMART goals and plans

Movement Activity: Movement Exploration

The following activity involves movement with three distinct goals: grounding, reaching, and expanding. Each activity includes three sequence options. You can choose the option that is most accessible to your body on a daily basis, or try all three to compare. Several of the sequences contain *asanas,* or yoga poses, which constitute one of yoga's eight limbs. We worked on *pranayama,* or breathing exercises, in the first chapter. In a way, we practiced *yama* (moral vows) and *niyama* (personal duties) through our exercises and readings. It's now time to put it all together with movement!

There is no right or wrong approach to these movement snacks. For example, you can perform the movements only once, but slowly and with long holds, or you can perform them several times at a quicker pace. Whichever approach you choose, set aside time to explore one sequence at a time and examine how you feel during, directly after, and the next day. Also, once you've gotten used to the sequences, think about how you can decrease the demands or increase the intensity to better meet your needs.

You can visit my website at www.MovementforEveryBody.org to find videos that accompany these instructions.

What you will need for this activity:

- Paper and pen or note-taking phone app

- Peaceful and comfortable space

- Fifteen to thirty minutes of dedicated time

- Optional mirror or phone to record video for feedback

INSTRUCTIONS

1. Set up a comfy area to perform upright movements (whether sitting or standing), or lie down on the floor or a bed to do the movements.

2. If possible, use a phone or mirror for visual feedback.

3. Try two to three attempts of the movement as instructed.

4. Take notes on how each part of the movement made you feel.

Grounding

Grounding Exercises: Option A Standing

1. Stand in a comfortable position in front of a sturdy chair.

2. Place your limbs on your hips or behind your head, or cross your arms across your chest.

3. Inhale, arch backward, expand your chest, and look up for Standing Cow Pose.

4. Exhale, curl forward, bring your chin to your chest, and look toward your belly button for Standing Cat Pose.

5. Inhale and stand normally. Then exhale, lean forward, place your limbs on the seat of the chair, look toward your belly button, and stand with feet shoulder width apart for Downward-Facing Dog.

6. Inhale and hold the position. Exhale while lowering knees to the floor for a tall kneeling position.

7. Inhale and stand tall on your knees. Exhale and bring the right foot forward for Low Lunge Pose.

8. Inhale and twist from this position. Keep the right limb on the chair or your hip, or reach it toward the sky. Exhale and return to center.

9. Repeat this cycle with the left leg.

PRO TIPS

- This exercise can be performed with or without the chair.

- Feel free to soften the floor with extra blankets under the knees.

- The legs can be about hip distance apart or wider for comfort.

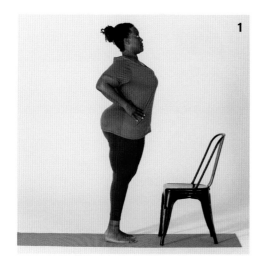

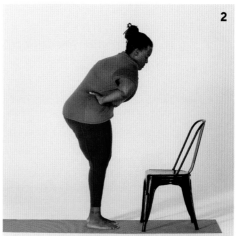

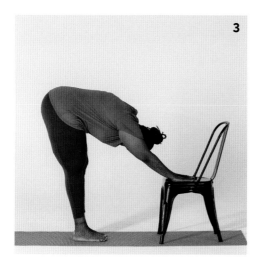

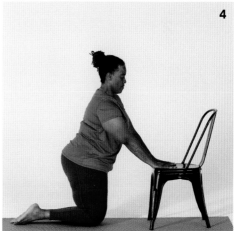

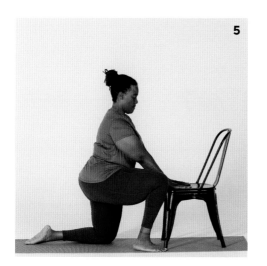

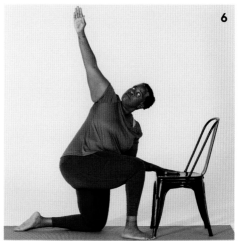

Grounding Exercises: Option B Seated

1. Sit upright on an armless chair, bench, firm bed, or sofa, with a sturdy table or chair placed in front of you.

2. Inhale, arch backward, expand your chest, and look up for Seated Cow Pose.

3. Exhale, curl forward, bring your chin to your chest, and rest your arms on the surface in front of you for Seated Cat Pose.

4. Inhale and sit upright, then exhale.

5. Inhale and place the right leg on a step stool or yoga block; exhale here.

6. Inhale and twist from this position, resting the left arm on your right thigh and right arm at your hip or reaching behind you. Exhale and return to center.

7. Repeat this cycle with the left leg.

PRO TIPS

- This exercise can be performed with or without the chair in front and with or without back support.

- Feel free to use your hands to help lift the leg whenever needed.

- The legs can be about hip distance apart or wider for comfort.

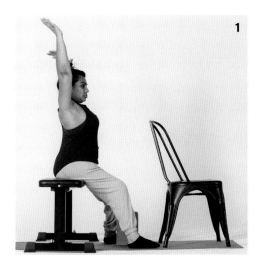

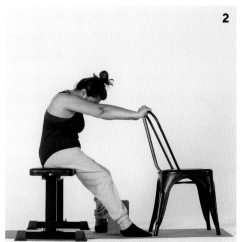

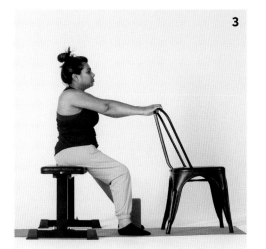

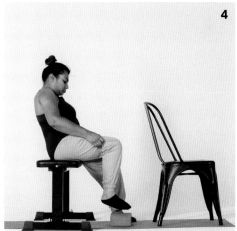

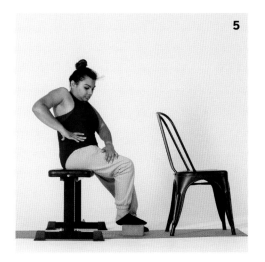

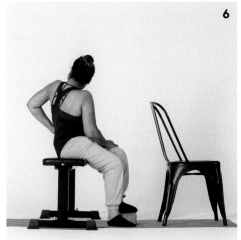

Grounding Exercises: Option C Lying Down

1. Lie down in a comfortable position on your back, with the knees bent.

2. Inhale, arch away from the floor, and expand your chest.

3. Exhale, press your lower back into the floor, and flatten your chest.

4. Inhale and bring the right leg toward your chest.

5. Exhale and twist by lowering the right leg to the left.

6. Inhale and return to starting position.

7. Repeat this cycle with the left leg.

PRO TIPS

- This exercise can be performed with a block or pillow to support the leg during the twist.

- Feel free to use the hands to help lift the leg whenever needed.

- If the twist is uncomfortable, lower the knee to create more space.

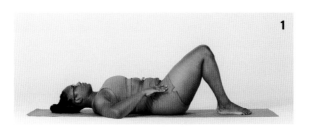

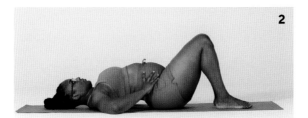

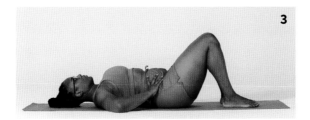

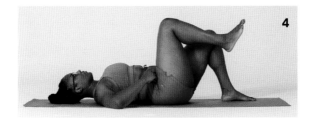

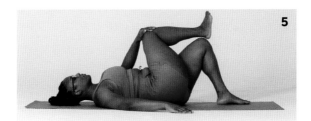

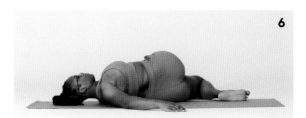

Reaching

Reaching Exercises: Option A Standing

1. Stand in a comfortable position, with feet together or apart.

2. Inhale, then exhale and lower down into Utkatasana (Chair Pose) as your arm reaches back.

3. Inhale and reach arms overhead as you stand on tiptoes.

4. Exhale and lower back down to normal standing position.

5. Inhale, and with the feet apart, rotate the right leg outward.

6. Exhale and reach down the right leg for Trikonasana (Triangle Pose).

7. Inhale and return to standing position. Exhale and rotate the right leg back to starting position.

8. Inhale, and with the feet apart, rotate the left leg outward.

9. Exhale and reach down the left leg for Trikonasana (Triangle Pose).

10. Inhale and return to standing position. Exhale and rotate the left leg back to starting position.

PRO TIPS

- This exercise can be performed while holding a chair, wall, or table if you need balance support.

- For the top arm in Triangle Pose, you can rest the hand on the hip or reach toward the ceiling.

- For the bottom arm in Triangle Pose, reach for the thigh, the shin, a chair, a step stool, or the floor.

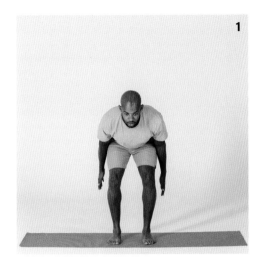

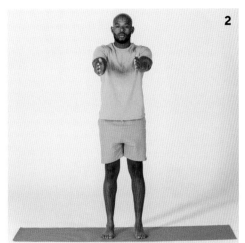

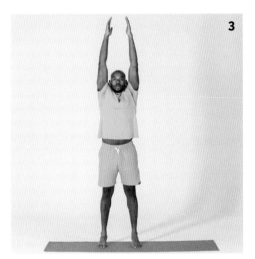

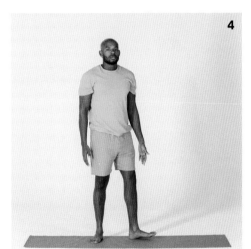

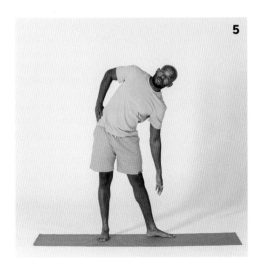

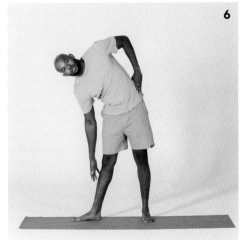

Reaching Exercises: Option B Seated

1. Sit upright on an armless chair, bench, firm bed, or sofa. The legs and/ or feet can be together or apart.

2. Inhale, then exhale as you reach the arms back and press the legs into the floor for Seated Utkatasana (Chair Pose).

3. Inhale and reach the arms overhead as you lift the heels off the floor.

4. Exhale and lower the arms back down to normal sitting position.

5. Inhale, and with the feet apart, rotate the right leg outward.

6. Exhale and reach down the right leg for Trikonasana (Triangle Pose).

7. Inhale and return upright. Exhale and rotate right leg back to starting position.

8. Inhale, and with the feet apart, rotate the left leg outward.

9. Exhale and reach down the left leg for Trikonasana (Triangle Pose).

10. Inhale and return upright. Exhale and rotate left leg back to starting position.

PRO TIPS

- This exercise can be performed with a block or step stool under both legs for Chair Pose.

- If there is a limb difference, a yoga block or step stool can help during Triangle Pose.

- For the top arm in Triangle Pose, you can rest it on the hip or reach toward the ceiling. For the bottom arm, reach for the thigh, the shin, a chair, a step stool, or the floor.

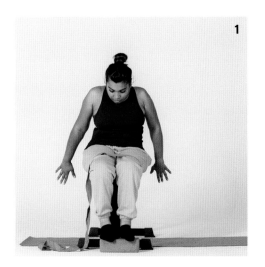

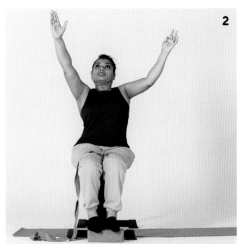

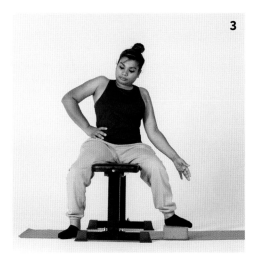

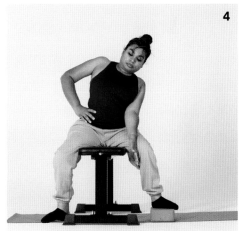

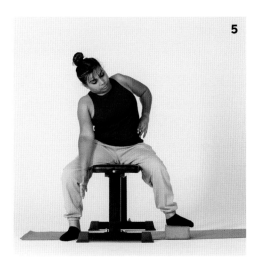

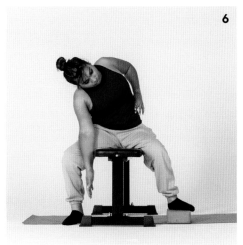

Reaching Exercises: Option C Lying Down

1. Lie down in a comfortable position on your back, with the knees bent and arms at your side.

2. Inhale, then exhale as you reach the arms overhead and press the legs into the floor to lift your bottom as high as you can for Setu Bandha Sarvangasana (Bridge Pose).

3. Inhale, then exhale as you lower back to starting position.

4. Inhale, and with the legs apart, rotate the right leg outward.

5. Exhale and reach down toward the right leg for a floor version of Trikonasana (Triangle Pose).

6. Inhale and return upright. Exhale and rotate right leg back to starting position.

7. Inhale, and with the legs apart, rotate the left leg outward.

8. Exhale and reach down the left leg for a floor version of Trikonasana (Triangle Pose).

9. Inhale and return upright. Exhale and rotate left leg back to starting position.

PRO TIPS

- This exercise can be performed with or without the arm movement during Bridge Pose. You can also add lifting heels off the floor once Bridge Pose is completed.

- For Triangle Pose, the arm on the same side as the rotated leg reaches down toward the thigh, shin, or foot. The opposite arm can rest on the hip or reach overhead.

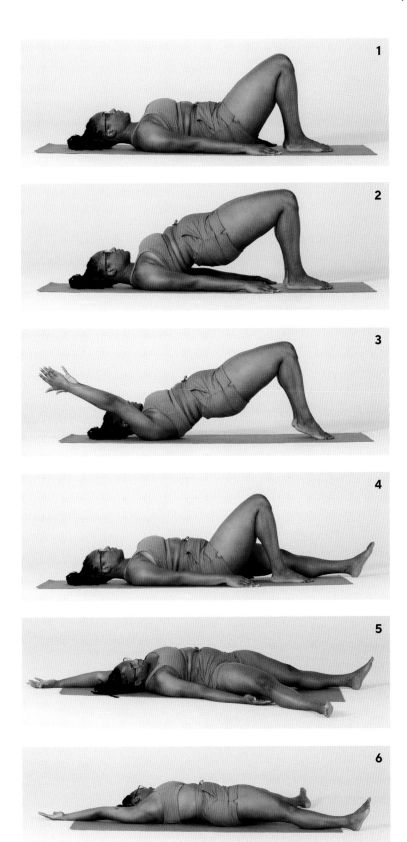

Expanding

Expanding Exercises: Option A Standing

1. Stand in a comfortable position in front of a sturdy chair.

2. Inhale to bend the right knee to bring your lower leg toward your bottom.

3. Exhale to rotate and swing the leg around to rest on the chair.

4. Inhale and place the hands on the the hip, thigh, or chair.

5. Exhale to squeeze the shoulder blades together as you lift the arms and bend them at the elbows.

6. Inhale, then exhale to lower the arms.

7. Inhale, then exhale to lower the leg.

8. Repeat this cycle with the left leg.

PRO TIPS

- This exercise can be performed with one arm, both arms, or neither resting on the chair for support.

- Feel free to play around with different heights by choosing a chair, step stool, or coffee table.

- Try to keep a slight bend in the knee of the standing, supporting leg.

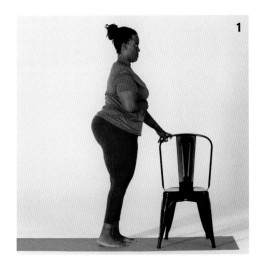

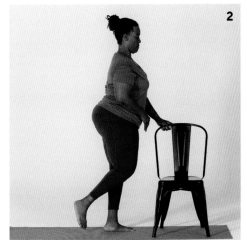

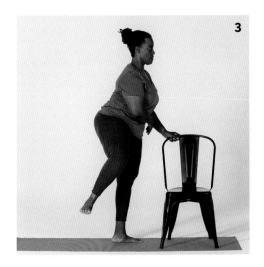

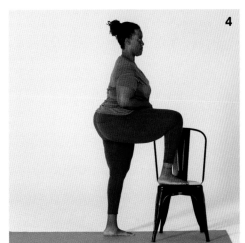

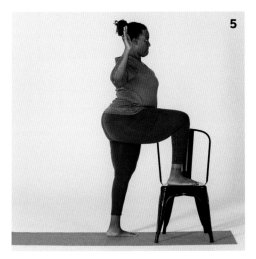

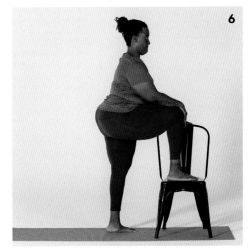

Expanding Exercises: Option B Seated

1. Sit in a comfortable position on an armless chair or bench or the edge of a bed, with a sturdy chair in front of you.

2. Inhale to slide the right foot back as far as you can.

3. Exhale to rotate and swing the leg around to rest on a block or stack of books.

4. Inhale, then exhale to squeeze the shoulder blades together as you lift the arms and bend them at the elbows.

5. Inhale, then exhale to lower the arms.

6. Inhale, then exhale to lower the leg.

7. Repeat this cycle with the left leg.

PRO TIPS

- This exercise can be performed with one arm, both arms, or neither resting on the chair for support.

- Feel free to play around with different heights by lifting the leg to more blocks or a higher step stool.

- Try to keep the sitting posture upright, with a neutral pelvis.

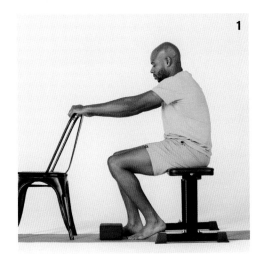

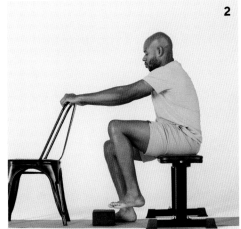

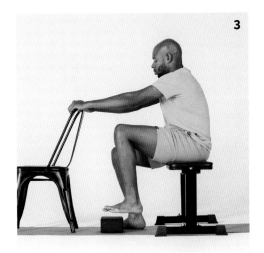

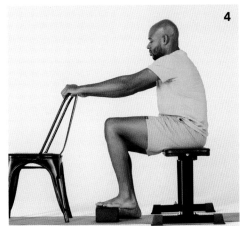

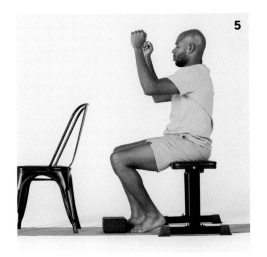

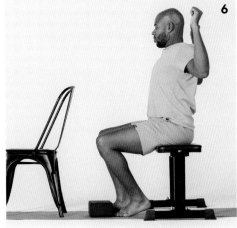

Expanding Exercises: Option C Lying Down

1. Lie down on your left side in a comfortable position, with both legs slightly bent.

2. Inhale to bend the right knee so the lower leg moves toward your bottom.

3. Exhale to rotate and swing the leg around to rest on a block or book in front of you.

4. Inhale, then exhale to swing the leg back to the starting position.

5. Move the block or book away from your body.

6. Inhale and exhale as you roll onto your belly and place your elbows by your chest.

7. Inhale, then exhale as you peel your upper body away from the floor for Bhujangasana (Cobra Pose).

8. Inhale and lie back down. Exhale and turn to lie down on your right side.

9. Reposition the block and repeat the cycle with the left leg.

PRO TIPS

■ This can be performed with a pillow or block placed under the head or anywhere else needed to increase comfort while lying down on your side.

■ Feel free to add cushioning or supports under the chest or belly while lying face down.

■ Feel free to tuck the toes for Cobra Pose, or to lay the feet flat.

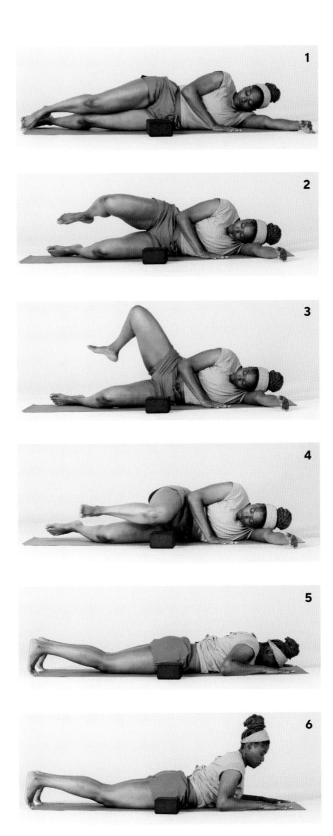

Enjoy

enjoy verb
en·joy in-ˈjȯi
to take pleasure or satisfaction in

Why Does Joyful Movement Matter?

We're in the home stretch of this inclusive fitness guide for better movement. We've appraised the values that keep us stuck, assessed all the variables we can and can't control, and explored how our bodies move. It's time to focus on enjoyment! The path to joy is also a path of liberation and an act of resistance. In finding joy we heal ourselves and resist systems of oppression. This is no small feat. Take a moment to pat yourself on the back for making it this far. Take a breath of gratitude for the work you've put in to move wholly and fully as a human being that deserves to exist on this Earth. You've done well!

It was super important for us to understand the big picture—how to set ourselves up for success, our body's strengths and weaknesses, and the goals we want to work on. With these foundations in place, we can finally direct our focus to the small details that will make all the difference in finding joyful movement that fulfills the body and mind.

What Makes Our Bodies Happy?

Joyful movement is all about fun and exploration, but there are still physical demands and foundational needs to consider. We've talked about variables to consider outside the moment of movement, such as sleep and nourishment; but what can we do while moving to keep our bodies happy?

The Warm-Up

Before getting to the main idea of any workout, movement, or other physical activity, a good warm-up can make all the difference in preparing your body and mind for the motion. The warm-up is the period of time when you move at a super-easy intensity for five to fifteen minutes before starting the workout. This period of time also serves as a transition point—a liminal space, if you will—that allows for mental check-in as well as physical check-in. As you warm up, you can let go of stressors that plagued you moments ago and focus on the movement ahead. As you move around, you can check in with your body and see how everything feels. The only tricky part of the warm-up is that one person's warm-up routine can be another person's entire workout. Whether it's a whole workout or a simple warm-up depends on the demands of the movement and the body that shows up that day. Choose movements that are gentle and low intensity compared to the activity planned, with respect to your ability and capacity. Of course, even if you've warmed up, that doesn't mean you jump straight into the maximal effort of the activity planned. You still need to take time to ramp up the intensity of the activity itself.

Here are a few examples of warm-ups before exercises:

- Gentle stationary cycling for five minutes before starting barbell squats

- Slow arm circles and trunk rotation before using a rowing machine

- Side lunges and heel raises before starting an outdoor hike

A Focus on Safety

While working out, a focus on safety can help to keep you connected to your body and chasing that joy. In terms of safety, be sure that your clothing and footwear suit the activity. Your options may be limited by funds and access, but do your best to choose clothing and footwear that are safe and comfortable. When making these choices, consider the demands of the activity and your sensory needs. For example: Are you tripping over your laces? Is the shirt tag aggravating you? Are you tired of pulling down your shorts? Do your feet hurt when you're done?

Exercise safety also includes the environment. Again, your options may be limited by funds and access, but do your best to move in an environment that makes you feel safe and welcomed. Engaging with joyful movement can be tough when an unsafe, toxic, or hostile environment pushes you into a hyperaroused fight-or-flight state. The other aspects of the environment are setup, space, and layout. This applies to all dedicated exercise spaces, whether you're at home or in someone else's space.

Here are a few tips to keep you safe while exercising:

- Limit fall hazards on the floor, such as cords, rugs, and small items.

- Any items on the floor should be a different color so that the contrast makes the obstacle clear.

- Limit use of gripless socks without shoes on slick surfaces where sliding is possible.

- Ensure there's enough space around the workout area to move around without bumping into anything.

- If exercising near stairs, ledges, curbs, or other uneven surfaces, make sure there is good lighting.

- Set up near a sturdy chair, wall, or handrail if you know you might need more support and balance for the activity.

Lots of Good Hydration

While exercising, we must also remember to properly hydrate. There is no universal recommendation for hydrating during exercise and movement. What your body requires may differ from others, and it may differ based on the intensity of the exercise. It can take some trial and error to figure out what your body requires for hydration and when. It also calls for paying close attention to how you feel before, during, and after the workout, as well as how much fluid you can tolerate in your stomach while moving around. For example, thanks to reflux I won't drink any liquids before lying down on my back to do bench presses. This means I have to be more attentive to hydrating appropriately before doing bench presses and after I'm finished with them. It can be helpful to start with blanket advice, as long as we bear in mind that blanket advice is general advice that doesn't take into consideration your specific needs.

Here are a few starting points to explore:

- Hydrate with water before the workout.

- Hydrate with water for low-intensity workouts.

- Consider adding drinks with carbohydrates *and/or* electrolytes for higher-intensity workouts, regardless of duration, such as Gatorade, Pedialyte, coconut water, Liquid IV, or Body Armor.

- Consider adding drinks with carbohydrates *and/or* electrolytes when exercising in hotter climates and environments.

- Consider adding drinks with carbohydrates and protein if you're unable to snack or eat a meal after higher-intensity workouts.

What Happens When It Hurts?

How do we navigate pain when it comes to intentional or joyful movement? First we must understand what pain is and where it comes from. The International Association for the Study of Pain (IASP) defines pain as "an unpleasant sensory and emotional experience associated with, or resembling that associated with, actual or potential tissue damage." They state that pain is a subjective experience involving both biological and psychological factors; therefore, a person's report of pain should be respected. The IASP also notes that pain (a subjective experience) and nociception (nervous system response triggered by potential damage) are not the same. This means the experience of pain is not a simple one and varies from person to person. Although pain is complicated, verbal descriptors can help us to decide how to respond to the experience.

Generally speaking, pain can be categorized and defined in many ways. Here we will chunk pain into categories of neurogenic (nerve), vascular (veins and circulation), inflammatory (can occur with other categories of pain), mechanical (muscles, bones, soft tissues), and non-nociceptive (no presence of damage).

Neurogenic pain is produced or generated by the nerves. Neuropathy is the term for unpleasant sensations resulting from damage to the nervous system, which often causes neurogenic pain. Nerve pain happens when a nerve is pinched, crushed, stretched, or damaged from trauma (e.g., falls, cuts), inflammation (e.g., autoimmune issues, pregnancy, poisoning, diabetes), or orthopedic events (e.g., overuse injuries, strains). Nerve pain can feel like pins and needles, a weird sensation of numbness or a body part being "asleep," itching, feelings of hot or cold liquid when you're not touching anything, or even buzzing. This type of pain may or may not change with position and activity. Nerve pain can be diagnosed and treated by a physical therapist or a neurologist. Depending on the situation, surgery may be needed, the condition may be temporary, exercises may help, or you might need medication. Depending on the cause, nerve pain can be managed with medication, physical therapy, heat or ice packs, transcutaneous electrical nerve stimulation (TENS), interferential current stimulation (IFS), acupuncture, anti-inflammatory teas and foods, supplements, and avoiding certain fabrics or textures.

Vascular pain is produced or generated by circulatory vessels. Vascular pain happens when there are issues with blood flow due to vascular disease (can be caused by autoimmune issues, pregnancy, injury, trauma, or diabetes) or unfortunate events such as blood clots and aneurysms. Vascular pain can feel like throbbing, a deep ache, heaviness, or fullness. This type of pain can change with position and activity. Vascular pain can be diagnosed and treated by a vascular surgeon. In emergent/red-flag situations where pain is intense or accompanied by other symptoms such as nausea and vomiting, a trip to urgent care or the ER may be warranted. For vein issues, compression and elevation decrease pain; but for arterial issues, compression and elevation can increase pain (i.e., compression socks are not for everyone!). Depending on the cause of vascular pain, medication or surgical intervention may be needed. It's important to note that vascular disease can also result in skin changes and skin ulcers.

Inflammatory pain is produced or generated by the presence of extra fluid or enlarged structures. Inflammation can be caused by trauma (e.g., falls, cuts), systemic issues or disease (e.g., autoimmune conditions, pregnancy, poisoning, diabetes), or orthopedic events (e.g., overuse injuries, strains). The presence of inflammation can also trigger nerve and vascular pain as fluid builds up and swollen tissues push against nerves and vascular tissues. Inflammatory pain may feel like a steady, constant fullness, dullness, heaviness, and throbbing. This type of pain does not usually change with position and activity. If you have had a recent injury or problem with muscles or joints, inflammation pain can be diagnosed and treated by an orthopedic doctor or physical therapist. If you are pregnant, the pain can be diagnosed and treated by an OBGYN. If neither of these things applies, consider an assessment with a physical therapist to rule out other causes, as well as a trip to a primary care provider for their recommendations on specialist referrals.

Mechanical pain is produced or generated by joints and their surrounding muscles and tissues. This includes tendons, cartilage, ligaments, bursa, menisci, labrum, and bones. Mechanical pain can be triggered by acute, or recent, causes (e.g., traumatic accident, slips, falls, injury) or chronic, or ongoing, causes (e.g., overuse injury, positions, imbalances). Acute mechanical pain can feel sharp, constant, or throbbing, since inflammation is more prominent. Chronic mechanical pain can feel dull and intermittent in comparison. Mechanical pain can feel deep or shallow, depending on structures involved. This type of pain usually changes with position and activity. Mechanical pain can be diagnosed and treated by an orthopedic doctor or physical therapist. Depending on the cause, treatment may involve prescribed exercise, medication, supplements, heat, ice, surgery, TENS, IFS, acupuncture, or lifestyle changes.

Non-nociceptive pain is produced or generated by the same sensory pathways in the absence of tissue damage. You might have seen the term "psychogenic pain," but this term is no longer used because it insinuates that the pain is "all in your head." Non-nociceptive pain is still real pain. This type of pain may or may not change with position and activity. It can feel like any of the above types of pain, which makes it harder to treat. For example, it can be an acute pain from an injury worsened by anxiety and depression, or it could be persistent pain related to chronic regional pain syndrome. This type of experience requires a care team that can help problem-solve the issues. This may include providers such as a neurologist, a physical therapist, a primary care provider, or an orthopedist.

You'll find a quick summary of different types of pain on the next page.

Navigating Pain with Exercise

We can still enjoy movement with pain, but we do need to be mindful of whether pain is cause for stopping the exercise. The experience of pain can vary across individuals and for the same individual with different variables. Don't let the possibilities overwhelm you with so much fear that you avoid movement entirely. Instead, use your curious mind to ask questions and explore options.

TYPE OF PAIN	CAUSES	DESCRIPTION	CONSTANT OR INTERMITTENT	CHANGE WITH POSITION	CHANGE WITH ACTIVITY	TREATMENT PROVIDERS	TREATMENT OPTIONS
Neurogenic	Nerve damage	Pins, needles, itching, shooting, pinching, buzzing, hot, cold, numbness	Both	No	Maybe	Neurologist, PCP, physical therapist	Physical therapy, heat, ice, electrical stimulation, medication, supplements, surgery, lifestyle changes
Vascular	Damage to blood flow	Fullness, heaviness, throbbing, deep aching	Intermittent	Yes	Yes	Vascular surgeon, PCP, physical therapist	Physical therapy, medication, supplements, surgery, compression garments
Inflammatory	Acute injury or chronic disease	Fullness, throbbing	Both	No	Maybe	PCP, OBGYN, rheumatologist, physical therapist, neurologist, massage therapist	Physical therapy, heat, ice, electrical stimulation, medication, surgery, lifestyle changes
Mechanical	Acute injury or chronic orthopedic problem	Sharp or dull ache, throbbing	Both	Yes	Yes	Orthopedist, physical therapist, massage therapist	Physical therapy, heat, ice, electrical stimulation, braces and splints, medication, supplements, surgery
Non-nociceptive	Any or none of the above	Any of the above	Both	Maybe	Maybe	Any of the above	Any of the above

Note: PCP = primary care provider.

Try this "traffic light method" the next time you experience pain with exercise:

 GREEN LIGHT: GO FOR IT! NO CHANGES REQUIRED. The pain is immediately gone when you stop doing the exercise, or the pain is a small ache, a twinge, or weird funky discomfort.

 YELLOW LIGHT: CAUTION. OBSERVE AND MODIFY. The mild pain continues after you stop moving, or the same exact mild pain is there at night or the next morning.

 RED LIGHT: STOP. The pain is excruciating during the exercise, or the pain is excruciating that night or the next morning.

We are not fragile beings. We don't need to fear movement, but we do need to do everything with intention. Intention means curiosity and observation. Try taking videos of yourself doing the movements or watching tutorials with different bodies for better form. Take note of any mental and physical demands that may be altering your exercise performance, and explore whether sleep or nourishment has affected your healing. Use this information to guide modifications for yellow-light pains and future plans for red-light pains. Modifications can include cutting down the intensity or the number of reps, or changing other exercise variables to give yourself more support.

Let's break down the traffic-light method with an example. Say you've been lifting weights in the gym and using the barbell for a couple of years, with a few tweaks and pings here and there but no serious injury. The weekend after a hiking trip, you return on Monday for kettlebell swings, lunges, and squats.

 GREEN LIGHT: You felt fine with swings, but you noticed a weird twinge with walking lunges and squats. Once you stop, the feeling is gone, and you can't pinpoint exactly where or when it bothers you. That night you wonder what the twinge was about, but by the next morning you nearly forget about it.

 YELLOW LIGHT: You felt fine with the swings but have pain with walking lunges and squats. The weird twinge is still there when you stop moving, so you decide to do more swings and walking carries instead of lunges and squats. That night the knee doesn't feel normal, and the next morning it's still a bit off. You review the past couple of days: Did you need an extra day of rest after hiking? Did anxiety about returning to work on Monday keep you up last night? For the next workout, you decide to work on static split squats instead of walking lunges and squats. You also touch your knee down onto a yoga block instead of going all the way to the floor, to limit the range of motion.

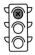 RED LIGHT: You feel okay with the swings but feel excruciating pain once you bend the knee deeply during walking lunges and squats. The pain isn't excruciating when you stop, but it's still achy. You decide to cut the leg workouts and head home. The next day it still hurts bad, so you rest and review the past few days: Did you wear bad shoes for hiking? Did you forget you kind of stepped weird on a shifting rock? Once the acute pain resolves, you test out movements without huge deep knee bends, then try light squats the next time, and finally resume normal activities if everything feels good.

How Can Options Foster Joy?

Throughout this book, there have been references to modifications, making choices (hello, agency!), and variations. As the journey comes to its end and you, my young grasshopper, prepare to take on the world, we must be sure that you understand exercise variations and how to make modifications on your own. To be clear, making these choices never equates to less ability or less worth. Many fitness professionals create content based on their own able-bodied perspectives, with limited training or experience in how different bodies move and require diverse options. So, seriously, stop feeling bad about it! Choosing a different workout, exercise modification, or variation that isn't shown doesn't make you any less of a person. If anything, it's self-care.

When it comes to exercise variations, it's helpful to understand the core aspects of all exercise and how they relate to your goals. One way to think about exercise is based on the FITT principle, developed by American College of Sports Medicine:

F = Frequency, or how often you exercise

I = Intensity, or how hard you exercise

T = Time, or how long you exercise

T = Type of exercise activity

The combination of all these principles can determine how you choose to move. For example, let's say you have this SMART goal: "In three months, I want to run at a moderate pace without getting out of breath." When making a SMART plan with the FITT principle in mind, you may choose to exercise once a week (frequency), at a moderate difficulty (intensity), for twenty minutes (time), by running at an outdoor park (type) because of access needs or recovery time needed. You could also choose to exercise daily (frequency), at a low difficulty (intensity), for five minutes (time), by stretching at home (type) because it's not that hard and doesn't require much effort or setup. The flexibility involved in choosing between these principles depending on the type of physical activity and your own SMART goals can be overwhelming! Remember, it's totally fine if you make a mistake and wind up overshooting or undershooting. There's a learning curve when applying principles on paper to your real life, which is never quite as simple as a textbook.

In addition to these principles, it can help to understand the terms *overload, specificity,* and *motor learning*.

- Overload: the exercise needs to be at a level above current capacity for a training effect to happen

- Specificity: the exercise needs to be specific to the activity or goal

- Motor learning: the exercise requires learning a new motor skill; with practice, the exercise can be performed efficiently

The combination of these principles can help us to understand the effects of exercise over time. For example, with the same SMART goal in mind, consider what would happen if the SMART plan included brisk walks three times a week. Would this provide enough overload? Well, that depends. The goal is to run at a moderate pace without getting out of breath, so if you get out of breath with a brisk walk, then yes, this activity provides enough overload. If walking at a brisk pace is a piece of cake, there will be no training effect from this activity, which means limited progress toward the goal. What would happen if the SMART plan included a rowing class once a week? Would this provide enough specificity? Probably not; you may get better endurance but this won't help your running form. What would happen if the SMART plan included treadmill running? This could help with motor learning if you used a mirror or recorded video to help with running form, since that would be harder to do while running outdoors.

Another set of terms that can help us make informed choices about move-ment denote the main types of exercise. Most exercise can be put into one of two categories: *anaerobic* or *aerobic*.

- Anaerobic exercise consists of movements that require short bursts of intense energy but do not use oxygen to break down glucose (sugar) to provide that energy, such as high-intensity interval training or weightlifting.

- Aerobic exercise includes movements that require longer bursts of energy and use oxygen to break down glucose (sugar) to sustain that energy, such as running or swimming

Either type of movement can result in muscle soreness. Generally speak-ing, starting new activities can cause more muscle soreness and much more rapidly—maybe even the same day. After doing the same exercises and types of movement over time, the way you experience soreness will usually change. Eventually some folks may experience only delayed-onset muscle soreness, which comes after one to three days, while other folks may experience no muscle soreness at all. In any case, the amount of soreness does not necessar-ily indicate whether progress is being made. We do not have to chase a certain feeling of soreness to feel a workout "counted," and we can understand that new movements and loads will probably make us more sore.

The final set of terms to help us make choices for how we move are *repe-tition, set,* and *rest intervals.* These variables can change the aim of a work-out to help us achieve different goals by providing different demands and intensity levels.

- Repetition (rep) = one completion of an exercise movement

- One-rep max (1RM) = the most you can do for a single repetition

- Set = one series of repetitions

- Rest = time spent in between sets

The combination of these variables can help us to achieve endurance, hypertrophy (muscle growth), power (the ability to overcome resistance over time), or strength (the ability to overcome resistance). These variables can be shifted and manipulated to plan both anaerobic and aerobic exercise to better suit our goals. See the table below for a general starting point for selecting reps, sets, and rest periods.

GOAL	INTENSITY	REPS	SETS	REST
Endurance	Low–medium	> 10	2–3	< 60 seconds
Hypertrophy	Medium	6–12	3–6	30–60 seconds
Power	Medium–high	< 6	2–6	2–5 minutes
Strength	Medium–high	< 3	3–5	2–5 minutes

For an anaerobic example of how to use this information, let's say you have this SMART goal: "In twelve weeks, I want to have a deadlift 1RM of 200 pounds." In this case, a selection of reps and sets intended to build power and/or strength would make the most sense. But if your SMART goal is "In twelve weeks, I want to deadlift 150 pounds more than ten times in one minute," a selection of reps and sets intended to build endurance and/or strength would make more sense.

With the above principles and terms in mind, it can be even easier to work on exercise variations and modifications in real time. The first step is to learn the "why"; then you can adjust the "how." Ask yourself: What is the main idea of the exercise, and at what point does the exercise stop working for you? Would it make sense to choose a variation of the exercise to achieve the goal? Or should you choose a modification to make the exercise (or program) more achievable?

Let's picture this SMART goal: "In twelve weeks, I want to squat 1RM of 150 pounds." You envision a conventional barbell squat for this goal, but when you try it, you find it hard to keep your knees from caving in at the very bottom. Don't despair; you have options! You could choose a variation such as a box squat or pin squats to avoid the very bottom and build strength from there. Or you could choose a modification, such as placing a light band around the thighs during warm-ups, to help your knees stay in line at the very bottom. You might even take note of whether it gets harder with fatigue and modify the reps to a lower amount before fatigue hits.

How Much Joyful Movement Do I Need?

As we chase joy and fulfillment with an embodiment practice, we might find ourselves asking: How do I know I'm doing enough? This can be a tough question to answer because it depends on the individual who's asking it. You may enjoy driving to the rock-climbing gym and training on a course three times a week, and that's more than enough. Or you might do that and also lift weights and attend virtual Zumba classes. It's entirely up to your access in terms of funds, mental demands, and physical capacity. I would say it's always smart to try only one new thing at a time, discern how much rest and recovery you need after doing the activity, and decide whether you actually like it before you add another movement practice to the mix. When we get to the journaling activity later, we'll dive into factors to consider when it comes to choosing movement.

The question of whether you're doing enough can also be tough to answer because we might not have even tried all the activities that bring joy, or we might be avoiding activities that we view as impossible to achieve. If the first scenario describes you, say less! See below for a list of different movement practices, and take note of anything that sounds new to you. If the second scenario describes you, say less yet again! See the "Resources" section at the end of this book for a list of educational organizations and databases that list fitness professionals to get you started on something new with confidence. And don't forget: it's okay to suck at something, it's okay to look silly, and it's definitely okay to fail. The point is having *fun*.

DIFFERENT MOVEMENT PRACTICES

- Weight training with dumbbells or kettlebells

- Barbell sports (powerlifting, weightlifting), bodybuilding, strongman

- Calisthenics, parkour, rock climbing (indoor or outdoor)

- Yoga: yin, *vinyasa, pranayama, hatha, ashtanga,* aerial

- Step, barre, Pilates (mat and reformer)

- Dance: Zumba, heels, chair dance, hip-hop, ballet

- Combat sports: boxing, Brazilian jiujitsu, kickboxing, fencing, wrestling

- Martial arts: karate, MMA, judo, kung fu, muay Thai, tae kwon do

- Ball sports: basketball, bowling, soccer, kickball, football

- Water sports: swimming, rowing, kayaking, surfing, water skiing, wakeboarding

- Aerial sports: lyra, aerial silks, bungee, suspension, pole dancing

- Cycling, rucking, hiking, running

- Stationary equipment: row machine, spin bike, air bike, recumbent bike, treadmill, StairMaster, elliptical

Journaling Activity: What Makes Me Happy

If you had a tough time in chapter 3 creating SMART goals based on joyful movement, this activity may help you develop your preferences for an embodiment practice. There are so many options and ways to move, which can be overwhelming to choose from when the toxic fitness default is often cardio for weight-loss purposes only. This activity can help to get the gears turning and hopefully steer you in the right direction to start trying some new moves.

What you will need for this activity:

- Paper and pen or note-taking phone app

- Peaceful and comfortable space

- Fifteen to twenty minutes of dedicated time

INSTRUCTIONS

1. Stand, lie down, or sit comfortably in any position.

2. Set up any sounds or smells that bring comfort.

3. Read the questions, then note your responses (they can be a few words or full sentences).

4. Consider recording audio or video answers if note-taking is not your jam.

QUESTIONS

- Do you prefer indoor or outdoor activities? What do you need for either?

- Do you like group activities, solo activities, or both? What helps you decide on this preference?

- Do you like having help, or do you prefer self-guided movement? If it depends, what does it depend on?

- Do you prefer live classes to be in person or virtual? What do you need for either?

- If financial access to an activity is a barrier, are there any public or community events that offer free or scholarship-based options?

- If physical access is a barrier, are there any options to change the environment or do it from home?

Movement Activity: Enjoy the Options

Your mission, should you choose to accept it, is to *have fun* with the final movement activity. Play with the variables we mentioned above paired with the movements below to see what you can come up with! This workout consists of three separate movement circuits, each with two options. After selecting an option, you will choose your own adventure by selecting the amount of time, number of reps, pace, and rest interval. Do you prefer the sensation of quick movements and a racing heart, or do you prefer slower motions and a lower heart rate? Are you a fan of holding poses, or do you despise counting so much that you avoid isometrics? Do you prefer continuous movement, or short bursts of movement with lengthier rest periods? Or maybe you try one round of exercise with strength gains in mind and see how it feels versus training with variables that support endurance gains.

You can visit my website at www.MovementforEveryBody.org to find videos that accompany these instructions.

What you will need for this activity:

- Paper and pen or note-taking phone app

- Peaceful and comfortable space

- Fifteen to thirty minutes of dedicated time

INSTRUCTIONS

1. Set up a comfy area to perform upright movements (whether sitting or standing), or lie down on the floor to do the movements.

2. If you can, set up a phone to record the movements, or position a mirror nearby.

3. Perform the movements as instructed with your chosen number of repetitions, pace, and rest time.

4. Take notes on how each part of the movement made you feel.

The Stand and Squat

Stand and Squat Option A

1. Stand upright with legs hip distance apart or wider.

2. Place a weight or weighted object at the inside of your left leg.

3. Inhale, bend forward, and reach down for the weight with your right arm.

4. Exhale and stand straight up as you bend the right arm to rest the weight near the shoulder.

5. Inhale, then exhale as you straighten the right arm, with the option of bending the upper body sideways to the left.

6. Inhale, stand straight up, and use both hands to hold the weight between your legs.

7. Exhale and lift the weight forward as you bend the knees as deeply as is comfortable into a squat.

8. Inhale to stand straight up. Exhale to place the weight at the inside of your right leg.

9. Repeat the cycle with the left arm.

PRO TIPS

■ If balance is an issue, try this sequence while leaning your back against a wall.

■ Feel free to use a lighter weight or skip the weighted object altogether.

■ Feel free to adjust the feet closer together or wider apart, with toes turned facing forward or toes turned outward.

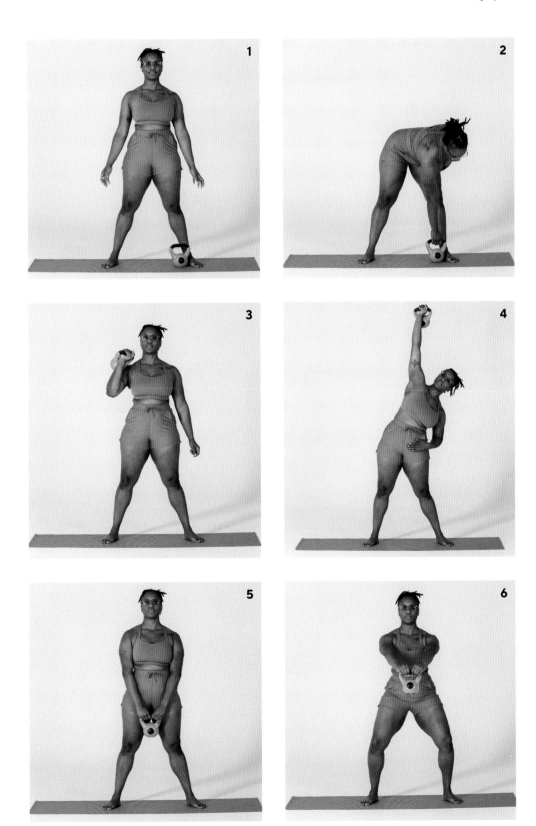

Stand and Squat Option B

1. Stand upright with legs hip distance apart or wider.

2. Inhale and reach both arms overhead as high as you can.

3. Exhale and lower both arms to the side, to shoulder height.

4. Inhale, then exhale as you reach the right arm toward the left thigh.

5. Inhale, then exhale as you reach the left arm toward the right thigh.

6. Inhale to stand straight up. Exhale to bend the knees as deeply as is comfortable into a squat.

7. Inhale and stand straight up, and reach both arms overhead as high as you can.

PRO TIPS

■ If balance is an issue, try this sequence while leaning your back against a wall.

■ You can hold a weighted object or place ankle weights on the arm for this sequence.

■ Feel free to adjust the feet closer together or wider apart, with toes turned forward or toes turned outward.

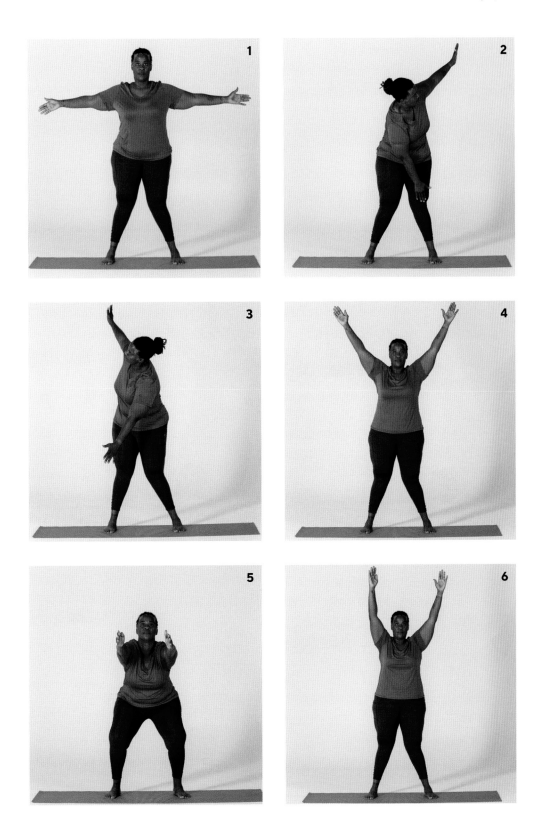

The Sit and Reach

Sit and Reach Option A

1. Sit upright on an armless chair, bench, firm bed, or sofa with legs wider than hip distance apart.

2. Place a weight or weighted object (filled water bottle, ball, etc.) at the inside of your right leg.

3. Inhale, bend forward, and reach down for the weight with your left arm.

4. Exhale and sit straight up as you bend the left arm to rest the weight near the shoulder.

5. Inhale, then exhale as you straighten the left arm, with the option of bending the upper body sideways to the right.

6. Inhale to sit straight up, then exhale to place the weight back down.

7. Repeat the cycle with the right arm.

PRO TIPS

■ If balance is an issue, try this sequence in a seat that has back support.

■ Feel free to use a lighter weight or skip the weighted object altogether.

■ Feel free to adjust the feet closer together or wider apart, with toes facing forward or toes turned outward.

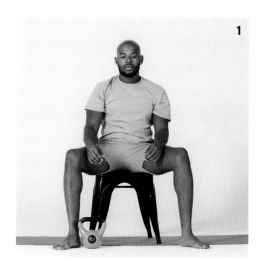

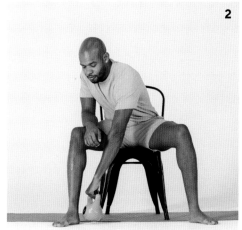

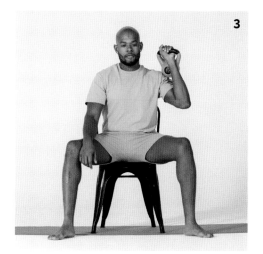

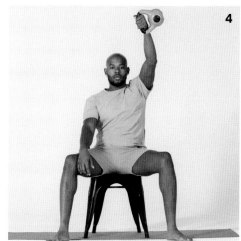

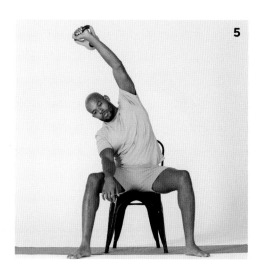

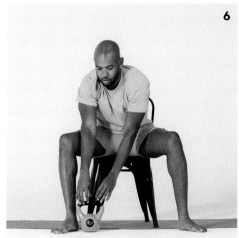

Sit and Reach Option B

1. Sit upright on an armless chair, bench, firm bed, or sofa with feet wider than hip distance apart.

2. Inhale, then exhale and twist to your left, placing the right hand on the left thigh and the left hand at your side or on your left hip.

3. Inhale and return to center. Then exhale and twist to your right, placing the left hand on the right thigh and the right hand at your side or on your right hip.

4. Inhale and return to center. Then exhale to lift the right arm overhead and bend sideways to the left.

5. Inhale and lower the arm. Then exhale to lift the left arm overhead and bend sideways to the right.

6. Inhale and lower the arm; then exhale as you sit upright.

7. Inhale and raise both arms to the side at shoulder level.

8. Exhale and bring the arms as close together as possible.

9. Inhale, drop the arms, and relax.

PRO TIPS

- If balance is an issue, try this sequence in a seat that has back support.

- You can hold a weighted object or place ankle weights on the arm for this sequence.

- Feel free to adjust the feet closer together or wider apart, toes turned facing forward or toes turned outward.

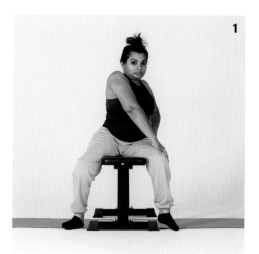

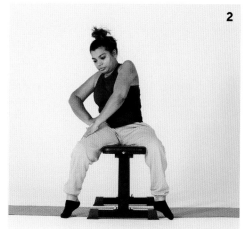

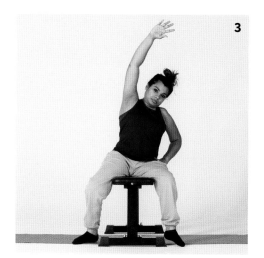

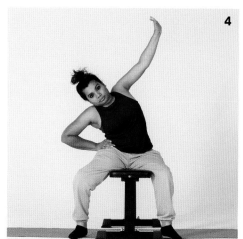

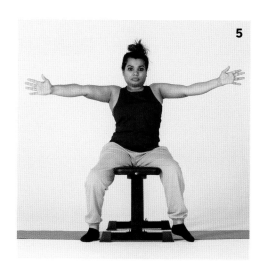

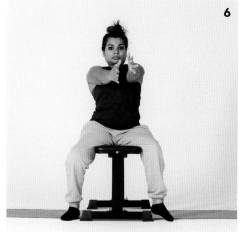

The Crunch and Hold

Crunch and Hold Option A

1. Lie down comfortably on your back, with the knees bent.

2. Place a weight or weighted object (filled water bottle, ball, etc.) on the floor above your head.

3. Inhale and reach both arms overhead to grab the weighted object.

4. Exhale and lift the weighted object over your chest.

5. Inhale, then exhale to reach the weight toward your left thigh.

6. Inhale to reset, then exhale to reach the weight toward your right thigh.

7. Inhale to rest, and bend your elbows to lower the weight to your chest.

8. Inhale, then exhale as you straighten the arms and lift the shoulders, feet, and head off the ground for a dead-bug hold.

9. Inhale in this position, then exhale to rest.

PRO TIPS

- You can always use a lighter weight or skip the weighted object altogether.

- Feel free to lift only the head, only the arms, or only the legs for the dead bug.

- Play around with resting the feet on pillows, a chair, or another surface for the whole sequence.

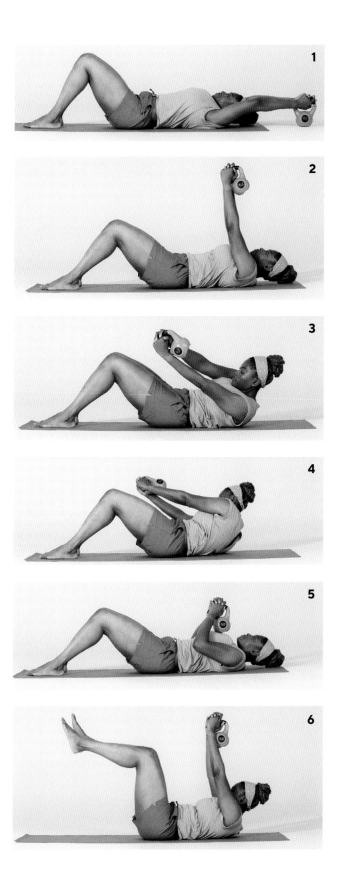

Crunch and Hold Option B

1. Lie down comfortably on your back with the knees straight.

2. Inhale, then exhale as you lift the left knee toward the chest and reach for the left knee with your right arm.

3. Inhale to rest, then exhale as you lift the right knee toward the chest and reach for the right knee with your left arm.

4. Inhale to lower the leg, then raise both arms together, clasping the hands if possible.

5. Exhale to twist and lower the arms to the right.

6. Inhale to return to center, then exhale to twist and lower the arms to the left.

7. Inhale to return to center, then exhale and rest the arms.

PRO TIPS

- You can hold a weighted object or place ankle weights on the arm or leg for this option.

- Feel free to bend the legs for more comfort during the twist.

- Feel free to add any blankets, cushions, or pillows under the head, back, knees, or ankles to add more comfort.

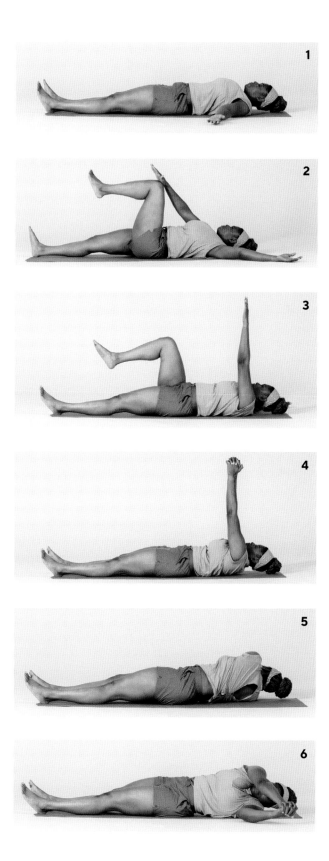

Resources

Online Educational Resources

Educational Resources for Neurodivergence

- Black Girl Lost Keys: www.blackgirllostkeys.com
- Neurodivergent Insights: www.neurodivergentinsights.com

Educational Resources for Movement Professionals

- Accessible Yoga School: www.accessibleyogaschool.com
- Black Girl Pilates: www.blackgirlpilates.com
- Body Positive Fitness Alliance: www.bodypositivefitness.com
- Coaches Corner kettlebell teaching course: www.liftoffstrength.ca/coaches-corner
- Coaching nontraditional athletes: www.rozthediva.com
- Creating affirming spaces e-book and guides: www.decolonizingfitness.com
- Embraced Body: www.embracedbody.com
- Fitness 4 All Bodies: www.fitnessforallbodies.com
- Hope Ignited trauma-informed training: www.hopeignitedtraining.com
- Tejal Yoga: www.tejalyoga.com/events
- Trauma Informed Weight Lifting: www.traumainformedweightlifting.com
- Yoga for All Bodies: https://yogaforallbodies.com/links/

Educational Resources for Movement Lovers

- Accessible Yoga Association: www.accessibleyoga.org

- Adaptive Training Foundation: www.adaptivetrainingfoundation.org

- Paige Fraser Foundation performing arts and wellness: www.thepaigefraserfoundation.org

- Disabled but Not Really adaptive health and wellness: www.disabledbutnotreally.org

- Disabled Girls Who Lift: www.disabledgirlswholift.com

- Disabled Hikers: www.disabledhikers.com

- Full Radius Dance: www.fullradiusdance.org

- Heidi Latsky Dance: www.heidilatskydance.org

- No Barriers USA: www.nobarriersusa.org

- Stopgap: www.stopgapdance.com

- Unlikely Hikers: www.unlikelyhikers.org

- WheelWOD adaptive fitness: www.wheelwod.com

Recommended Reading

- *Accessible Yoga: Poses and Practices for Every Body* by Jivana Heyman

- *Atomic Habits: An Easy & Proven Way to Build Good Habits & Break Bad Ones* by James Clear

- *Beyond Beautiful: A Practical Guide to Being Happy, Confident, and You in a Looks-Obsessed World* by Anuschka Rees

- *Big & Bold: Strength Training for the Plus-Size Woman* by Morit Summers

- *Body Aware: Rediscover Your Mind-Body Connection, Stop Feeling Stuck, and Improve Your Mental Health with Simple Movement Practices* by Erica Hornthal

- *The Body Is Not an Apology: The Power of Radical Self-Love* by Sonya Renee Taylor

- *The Body Liberation Project: How Understanding Racism and Diet Culture Helps Cultivate Joy and Build Collective Freedom* by Chrissy King

- *Deconstructing the Fitness-Industrial Complex: How to Resist, Disrupt, and Reclaim What It Means to Be Fit in American Culture* by Justice Roe Williams, Roc Rochon, and Lawrence Koval

- *Demystifying Disability: What to Know, What to Say, and How to Be an Ally* by Emily Ladau

- *Disability Visibility: First-Person Stories from the Twenty-First Century* by Alice Wong

- *Embrace Yoga's Roots: Courageous Ways to Deepen Your Yoga Practice* by Susanna Barkataki

- *Every Body Yoga: Let Go of Fear, Get On the Mat, Love Your Body* by Jessamyn Stanley

- *Fat Girls in Black Bodies: Creating Communities of Our Own* by Joy Arlene Renee Cox

- *Fearing the Black Body: The Racial Origins of Fat Phobia* by Sabrina Strings

- *Lifting Heavy Things: Healing Trauma One Rep at a Time* by Laura Khoudari

- *A Queer Dharma: Yoga and Meditations for Liberation* by Jacoby Ballard

- *Set Boundaries, Find Peace: A Guide to Reclaiming Yourself* by Nedra Glover Tawwab

- *The Slow AF Run Club: The Ultimate Guide for Anyone Who Wants to Run* by Martinus Evans

- *Tough: Building True Mental, Physical & Emotional Toughness for Success & Fulfillment* by Greg Everett

- *Yoga Where You Are: Customize Your Practice for Your Body and Your Life* by Dianne Bondy and Kat Heagberg Rebar

Databases Listing Fitness Professionals

- *Database of Affirming Fitness & Movement Practitioners* (free) by Decolonizing Fitness: www.decolonizingfitness.com/products /affirming-database-of-fitness-movement-specialist

- *Find a Trauma Informed Personal Tainer* by Hope Ignited: www.hopeignitedtraining.com/directory

- *Trauma Informed Practitioners* by Trauma Informed Weight Lifting: www.tiwl.org/community

- *Workout Database* by Lauren Leavell Fitness and Nonnormative Body Club: www.laurenleavellfitness.com/fitnessdatabase

Bibliography

American College of Sports Medicine. *ACSM's Guidelines for Exercise Testing and Prescription*. 10th ed. Philadelphia: Wolters Kluwer, 2018.

Ellis, Philip. "See if You Have Enough Balance to Pass This Simple 60-Second 'Old Man Test.'" *Men's Health,* November 27, 2021. https://www.menshealth.com/fitness/a38365792/chris-hinshaw-chris-bell-60-second-old-man-test/.

Miserandino, Christine. "The Spoon Theory Written by Christine Miserandino." But You Don't Look Sick, n.d. Accessed January 1, 2023. https://butyoudontlooksick.com/articles/written-by-christine/the-spoon-theory/.

National Human Genome Research Institute. "Eugenics and Scientific Racism." May 18, 2022. https://www.genome.gov/about-genomics/fact-sheets/Eugenics-and-Scientific-Racism.

Neff, Megan A. "Welcome to the Neurodivergent Insights Resource Page." Neurodivergent Insights, n.d. Accessed January 1, 2023. https://neurodivergentinsights.com/resources.

Office of Disease Prevention and Health Promotion. "Social Determinants of Health." Healthy People 2030, n.d. Accessed December 15, 2023. https://health.gov/healthypeople/priority-areas/social-determinants-health.

Office of Equity, Vitality, and Inclusion, Boston University Chobanian and Avedisian School of Medicine, Boston Medical Center, and Boston University Medical Group. "White Supremacy." *Glossary for Culture Transformation,* 2021. https://www.bmc.org/glossary-culture-transformation/white-supremacy.

Parker, Ilya. "What Is Toxic Fitness Culture?" Decolonizing Fitness, June 17, 2020. https://decolonizingfitness.com/blogs/decolonizing-fitness/what-is-toxic-fitness-culture.

Rahman, Mahbubur, Jeff R. Temple, Carmen Radecki Breitkopf, and Abbey B. Berenson. "Racial Differences in Body Fat Distribution among Reproductive-aged Women." *Metabolism* 58, no. 9 (2009): 1329–37. https://doi.org /10.1016/j.metabol.2009.04.017.

Raja, Srinivasa N., Daniel B. Carr, Milton Cohen, Nanna B. Finnerup, Herta Flor, Stephen Gibson, Francis J. Keefe, et al. "The Revised International Association for the Study of Pain Definition of Pain: Concepts, Challenges, and Compromises." *PAIN* 161, no. 9 (2020): 1976–82. https://doi.org /10.1097/j.pain.0000000000001939.

Siegel, Daniel J. *The Developing Mind: How Relationships and the Brain Interact to Shape Who We Are.* 3rd ed. New York: Guilford Press, 2020.

Smith, Leah. "#Ableism." The Center for Disability Rights, n.d. Accessed January 1, 2023. https://cdrnys.org/blog/uncategorized/ableism.

Smith, Sean B., Jeffrey B. Geske, Thomas D. Keenan, Nicholas A. Zane, Jennifer M. Maguire, and Timothy I. Morgenthaler. "Morbid Obesity Is Associated with Delayed Diagnosis and Management of Acute Pulmonary Embolism." *CHEST* 138, no. 4 (2010): 936A. https://doi.org/10.1378 /chest.10150.

Index

italic page numbers indicate photos

Acknowledgments

I am forever grateful to be in community with folks who have shaped my personal journey with movement, enriched the exploration of my disability identity, and deepened my skill set as a movement professional. I want to thank Ilya Parker of Decolonizing Fitness, who was the first person I ever encountered speaking of toxic fitness culture and putting words to thoughts I didn't even know I had. Special thanks to Justice Roe, who engulfed me in his world of Fitness 4 All Bodies, which led me to learn and get connected with so many other professionals and health care providers who *actually* care. I am also grateful to Justice Roe, Roc Rochon, and Lawrence Koval for including me in their anthology, *Deconstructing the Fitness-Industrial Complex.* Many thanks to Accessible Yoga School, founded by Jivana Heyman and Amber Karnes, who allowed me to appreciate yoga's roots, incorporate accessibility in everything I do, and support yoga teachers who are doing the same. When I initially took a two-hundred-hour teacher training, I had so many visceral reactions to conversations that decentered the need for accessibility in a practice that has always been meant for every- and anyone. Lastly, my deepest gratitude to Marybeth Baluyot, the founder of Disabled Girls Who Lift, for being the springboard of embracing my disability pride and diving into the community. Of course, there are many more people I'm grateful for, and one page isn't enough to name them all. To all of my TikTok and Instagram besties, I am thankful for being seen and supported by all of you.

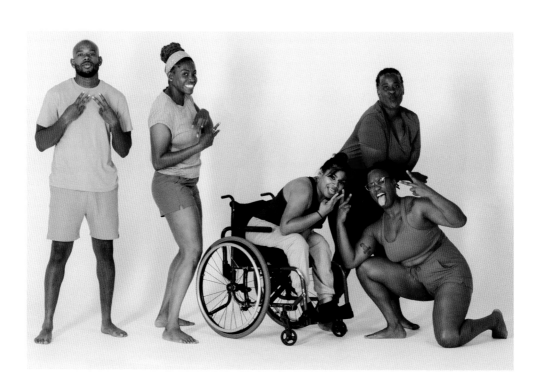

About the Author

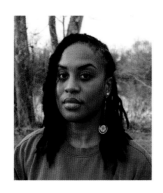

Dr. Marcia Dernie (she/they) is the child of Haitian immigrants who lives in Florida on Seminole land. They are a gender-fluid yoga teacher, physical therapist, disabled Black creative, and strength athlete with a chronic illness. She is the owner of Move With Marcia, which provides both free and affordable resources to help people move better through mobility exercises and yoga. Marcia also cohosts the @DisabledGirlsWhoLift podcast. You can connect with her on DoctorMarcia.com, and you can find her on Instagram, YouTube, and TikTok by searching for @MovewithMarcia.

About North Atlantic Books

North Atlantic Books (NAB) is an independent, nonprofit publisher committed to a bold exploration of the relationships between mind, body, spirit, and nature. Founded in 1974, NAB aims to nurture a holistic view of the arts, sciences, humanities, and healing. To make a donation or to learn more about our books, authors, events, and newsletter, please visit www.northatlanticbooks.com.